WALL PILATES WORKOUT FOR WOMEN

A 25-Day Illustrated Guide to a Full Body Transformation, Burning Belly Fat, and Building Your Core Strength + Nutritional Tips and Recipes.

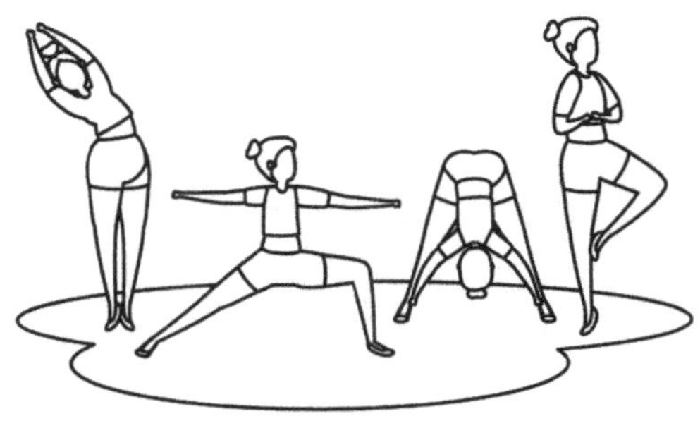

SAVANNAH USHER

Table of Contents

Introduction

Pilates has shown itself to be a timeless and successful strategy for achieving comprehensive well-being in the fitness industry, where trends come and go like the seasons. We're going to take it a step further now, or perhaps closer to the wall. Welcome to the exciting world of Wall Pilates, where the commonplace is transformed into the exceptional and your path to a stronger, healthier you takes on a fascinating twist.

Imagine engaging in physical exercise that not only changes your body but also uses a wall's stability and support. It's like having a trustworthy training partner in the convenience of your own home. Wall Pilates is a great option for women looking for a flexible and interesting workout routine because of its accessibility and simplicity.

Let's now prepare the ground for your journey into the Wall Pilates realm. First things first, set aside your prior knowledge of traditional Pilates for a bit. A dynamic twist that gives your practice a new depth is introduced by Wall Pilates. As we explore this method, you'll learn about the mutually beneficial relationship that exists between your body and the wall. This alliance opens up a world of exercises that target muscles you never even knew you had.

Prior to diving into the specifics, let's discuss why Pilates is a lifestyle rather than merely a workout regimen. Pilates isn't about working out for long hours or burning plenty of calories. It's a deliberate, thoughtful exercise that strengthens the bond between your body and mind. Furthermore, Wall Pilates enhances this mind-body connection by emphasizing deliberate placement against the wall and controlled movements, resulting in a harmonious combination of strength, flexibility, and mental clarity.

Think of the wall as your silent but reliable exercise buddy as you set out on this Wall Pilates adventure. It turns into the steadying influence that encourages you to push boundaries and redefine what your body is really capable of. Enjoy the feeling of every thoughtful movement instead of timing the remaining seconds in a set, and use the wall as a reference to balance and perfect form.

The benefits of Wall Pilates are not the only things that make it versatile. It's an acceptance of your individuality and a judgment-free celebration of your current fitness level. Whether you are an experienced Pilates practitioner or a beginner keen to learn more about this energizing form of exercise, the wall becomes a constant—a comforting presence that changes with you, providing support as you overcome obstacles and succeed in your workout.

Let's now dispel the misconception that Pilates is only appropriate for people looking for mild exercise. All fitness levels can benefit from wall Pilates, which adds a dynamic element that can be as hard or as soft as you like. The regulated intensity that gives you a sense of empowerment, both psychologically and physically, is just as important as the burn.

In the pages that follow, we'll reveal the mysteries of Wall Pilates and go over a wide range of exercises designed to tone your body, increase your energy, and improve your overall health. Prepare to rethink Pilates as the wall takes on the role of a painting showcasing your fortitude, resiliency, and self-awareness.

Without further ado, let's explore the world of Wall Pilates, which has the power to alter people. Here, a session is more than simply a physical exercise; it's an experience that nourishes your body, soothes your mind, and helps you live a happier, healthier life. Prepare to embrace the wall and start your Pilates journey!

CHAPTER 1: Understanding Wall Pilates

What is pilates?

Pilates can be compared to that sage, sympathetic buddy who helps you become a stronger, more self-aware version of yourself. Imagine a training regimen that nourishes your mind and spirit in addition to changing your physique. That's the essence of Pilates, an all-encompassing kind of exercise that has been molding people for almost a century.

Fundamentally, Joseph Pilates developed the mind-body technique known as Pilates in the early 1900s. Pilates was developed as a way to strengthen and heal the human body, and it has since spread throughout the globe as a popular, adaptable form of exercise.

Pilates is unique in that it emphasizes control, flow, and accuracy in its movements. It's about using your muscles with awareness and meaning, not just mindless repetitions. Imagine a sequence of purposeful, flowing movements that combine breath with movement to create a symphony of flexibility and strength.

The idea that your core is your body's powerhouse is fundamental to Pilates. A strong core is the cornerstone of a healthy body, according to Pilates. Your entire torso, from your pelvic floor to your shoulders, is made up of muscles that work together to form the powerhouse, not just your abs. Pilates sculpts your stomach and stabilizes and supports your entire body by using and strengthening these muscles.

Because of their adaptability, Pilates movements are suitable for people of all fitness levels. Pilates can be customized to accommodate your specific needs, regardless of your level of experience or where you are in your fitness journey. Your workouts can be made more challenging and varied by employing specialist equipment like the reformer, which can be used with your body weight or on a mat.

The integration of breath is one of the main principles of Pilates. According to Joseph Pilates, breathing correctly improves the effectiveness of movements by supplying the body with oxygen and energizing the blood. Breath is not an afterthought in Pilates exercises; rather, it is an essential component that synchronizes with your movement patterns.Pilates aims to create balance between strength and flexibility, not merely muscle growth. Traditional fitness regimens frequently overlook the value of flexibility in favor of concentrating only on strength training. To guarantee that your body moves with elegance and resiliency, Pilates creates a lovely balance by encouraging both strength and flexibility.

Pilates's versatility is what makes it so beautiful. Pilates can be tailored to your goals, whether they are to improve athletic performance, relieve back discomfort, or tone your muscles. Because of its mild impact, it is easy on the joints and appropriate for people of all ages.

Pilates fosters a mindful connection between your body and mind in addition to its physical benefits. The methodical motions and attention to breath produce a meditative atmosphere that provides a break from the daily grind. It's a time for self-care and self-discovery, not just exercise.

Pilates is essentially a discovery of your body's potential, a voyage of self-improvement, and a celebration of your individual strength. It's about living in the now, seeing the flow of every action, and valuing the amazing apparatus that is your body.

Thus, keep in mind that Pilates is a life-changing practice that goes outside the studio, impacting your movement, breathing, and eventually, your way of life, the next time you get out your mat or hop on the reformer. Introducing you to the world of Pilates: a complete approach to physical and mental well-being that benefits both the body and the spirit.

The Benefits of Pilates for Women

With its foundations in conscious movement, Pilates has become a potent ally for women who are looking for complete well-being. Pilates has other advantages that go beyond the physical, such as stronger, more flexible muscles and improved mental and emotional well-being. Now, let's explore the fascinating realm of Pilates and discover why it has grown to be a beloved exercise regimen for ladies worldwide.

Pilates is, above all, a celebration of strength. It is a sleek, sculpted strength that empowers women in their daily lives, not the huge, scary strength commonly associated with weightlifting. Pilates' methodical, controlled motions work several muscle groups at once, creating a balanced, harmonious body that leads to functional strength. Pilates gives women the power they need, naturally incorporated into their lives, whether they are hauling groceries, racing after little children, or tackling a demanding workday.

Flexibility is a key component in the pursuit of fitness, and Pilates excels in this area. Pilates exercises have a beautiful flow that stretches muscles and increases joint mobility. This increased flexibility helps with posture, lowers the chance of injury, and improves sports performance. The gift of greater flexibility is like a secret weapon for women juggling the demands of their personal and professional lives; it helps them to smoothly navigate life's curveballs.

Pilates celebrates the mind-body connection in addition to the physical, offering women a haven away from the stress of everyday life. Pilates promotes mental clarity and lowers stress levels through its emphasis on breath and mindfulness. Women find a priceless escape from the constant demands on their time and energy in the calm cocoon of a Pilates session. This mental renewal serves as the basis for resilience, empowering women to approach obstacles with composure and center.Pilates is unique in that it can be tailored to match different fitness levels and medical problems. Pilates extends a warm welcome to everyone, regardless of fitness level or time away from exercise. Because the focus is on regulated movements, women of various ages and fitness levels can begin with exercise in a calm and approachable manner. Pilates is also well known for its therapeutic advantages, helping with postpartum recuperation and offering relief from ailments like back discomfort. Because of its universality, Pilates serves as a supporting companion for women at all phases of their lives rather than merely a fitness regimen.

With its emphasis on longevity and sustainability, Pilates stands out among the many high-impact workouts and fast solutions available today. Each movement is certain to have meaning and impact since quality is prioritized over quantity. Pilates is about developing a long-lasting relationship with your body, not about getting results right away. This focus on mindful movement promotes a good body image in addition to preventing fatigue. Through Pilates, women connect with their bodies and gain a deep understanding of what they are capable of, which promotes acceptance and self-love.As social relationships are essential to general health, Pilates, which is frequently done in groups, fosters community. The common path of self-improvement forges relationships outside of the studio. Women who practice with other women find support and motivation from one another, fostering a community that celebrates each other's accomplishments, no matter how minor. The feeling of community that arises from these relationships enhances the Pilates experience, transforming it from a workout into a shared journey.

In conclusion, Pilates has several advantages for women that go well beyond its physical effects. It embraces community, sustainability, inclusivity, strength, flexibility, and awareness in a holistic way. Pilates turns into a safe refuge where women can take care of their emotional and physical health, creating a balanced, harmonious environment that permeates every aspect of their lives. Therefore, Pilates beckons with open arms, eager to reveal its many gifts, to any woman looking for a pleasant and transforming road to wellbeing.

Why Wall Pilates?

Wall Pilates is a novel and dynamic method to fitness and holistic well-being that fits in well with the lives of women looking for a well-rounded, efficient exercise program. This cutting-edge approach not only gives women a fresh lease on life and resilience, but it also meets their varied requirements in a way that is powerful and easily accessible.

Why Wall Pilates, then? Imagine the combination of classic Pilates exercises with the wall's support and resistance. It's a transformative experience that goes beyond the confines of traditional exercise regimens; it's not just a workout.

First and foremost, Wall Pilates gives people of all fitness levels a solid foundation. The wall is a trustworthy companion that will assist and mentor you during your Pilates adventure, regardless of your level of experience. This accessibility is revolutionary because it removes obstacles for people who previously might have been afraid or hesitant to begin a new exercise program.

Wall Pilates is unique in that it places a strong emphasis on core stability and strength. For women, having strong core muscles is essential to preserving general health and energy. With wall Pilates, you can precisely target these muscles and establish a strong foundation that will support and enhance all other parts of your fitness. Your core will get stronger and more engaged through a sequence of expertly designed motions, which will enhance your posture, balance, and midsection shape.

Wall Pilates offers your exercise regimen a contemplative and attentive component in addition to its physical advantages. Pilates focuses on the relationship between breath and movement, and the wall acts as a stabilizing element to strengthen this mind-body balance. Every breath and movement becomes deliberate as you press into the wall, clearing your mind and relieving tension.

We must not overlook Wall Pilates's usefulness. In a world where time is of the essence, this practice's simplicity is noteworthy. Neither a sizable dedicated space nor a variety of equipment are required. Your living room or office can be transformed into a haven for physical well-being with just one wall. Because of its accessibility, Wall Pilates may be easily incorporated into your everyday routine, transforming routine moments into chances for rest and renewal.

Since women frequently have to balance a lot of commitments, Wall Pilates' versatility is a real benefit. This approach honors the demands of your lifestyle, whether you're a stay-at-home parent, a busy worker, or someone with a demanding schedule. You may fit in a fast practice against the wall and feel your energy and vitality rising throughout the rest of the day.

Additionally, Wall Pilates promotes inclusivity and a sense of community. The practice's ease of sharing with friends and family creates opportunity for shared wellness experiences because of its simplicity. You'll experience a supportive and inspiring camaraderie with other participants as you press into the wall, making your fitness journey a shared experience.

Essentially, Wall Pilates is a comprehensive approach to health and self-discovery rather than just a physical exercise. It's about embracing a lifestyle that puts your health first, finding power in simplicity, and developing a mind-body connection. Why Wall Pilates, then? Because it invites you to reinvent what fitness means in your life and is a transforming, approachable, and empowering journey.

CHAPTER 2: Getting Started

Preparing Your Space

First, let's discuss the actual place. Locate a space in your house where you can stretch and move around comfortably. It doesn't have to be large; a spare corner in your living room or a designated area can do just as well. Make sure there are no risks or impediments, giving you a secure space to concentrate on the next exercise.

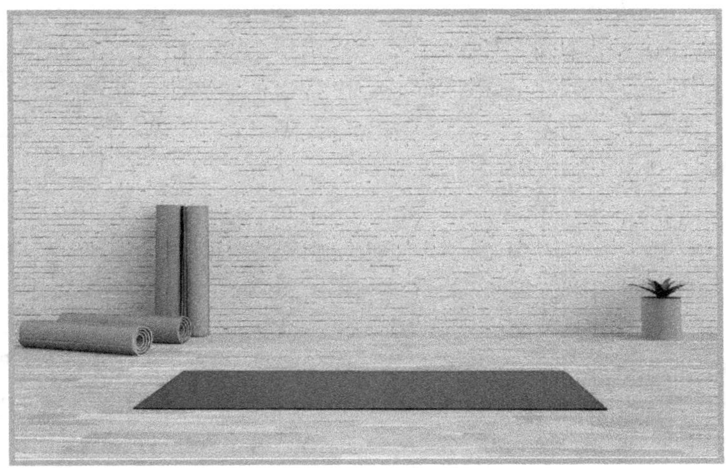

A spare corner in your house

Think about the floor underneath you. Even while Pilates is a low-impact workout, it can nevertheless benefit from a comfy surface. To soften your movements, use a yoga mat or a soft surface if at all possible. This gives your routine an extra layer of comfort while simultaneously supporting your body.

Let's now discuss the atmosphere in more detail. For Pilates classes, natural light might be your best friend. Pick an area with lots of natural light if at all possible. Let the sunshine in by opening the curtains or blinds; it will brighten the space and help you think positively.

Soft artificial lighting can create a comfortable atmosphere in situations when natural light is rare. To create a mood, think about utilizing lamps or movable lighting. A well-lit area improves your mood and makes it easier for you to observe your actions, which makes working out more pleasurable.

Let us now discuss the audio component. Pilates is no different from any other workout when it comes to the influence of music. Make a playlist of your best songs, preferably upbeat and rhythmic. Your motions will become more rhythmic and motivated with the correct music, which will improve the flow and enjoyment of the workouts.

If you want a more subdued atmosphere, think about using soothing instrumental music or sounds from nature. The idea is to create a space that feels right for you so that when you perform Wall Pilates, you may feel focused and at ease.

Let's now focus on the environment you are in. Clear the area. In addition to reducing distractions, a neat workspace encourages concentration and clarity of thought. Clear out any extraneous items and arrange your decor to create a visually appealing area that promotes focus and mobility.

Individual touches can have a big impact. Maybe you have a favorite plant, a quote that inspires you, or maybe a piece of art that motivates you. These accessories can bring a pleasant atmosphere to your training area that will improve your Pilates experience.

Let's now examine the technological aspect. Make sure all of your electronics are fully charged and operational. Having your gadgets ready reduces the possibility of interruptions throughout your workout, whether you're utilizing a fitness app or an internet video.

Recall that the idea is to design an environment that expresses your own style and inspires you to perform your Wall Pilates exercises on a regular basis. When you take the time to set up your training room, you're creating an atmosphere that promotes mental health and well-being as you progress through your fitness journey, not just a place to work out. Savor the procedure and allow your ready area to serve as the setting for your inspiring Pilates classes.

Essential Equipment

Before you start, let's chat about the essential equipment that will make your Wall Pilates workouts both effective and enjoyable.

The Wall: Your Main Support

Of course, a strong wall is your most important requirement. Select a level, unobstructed area where you may lean, sit, and execute different exercises without difficulty. Throughout the workout, the wall will be your dependable partner, providing stability for a variety of movements.

Yoga Mat or Exercise Mat

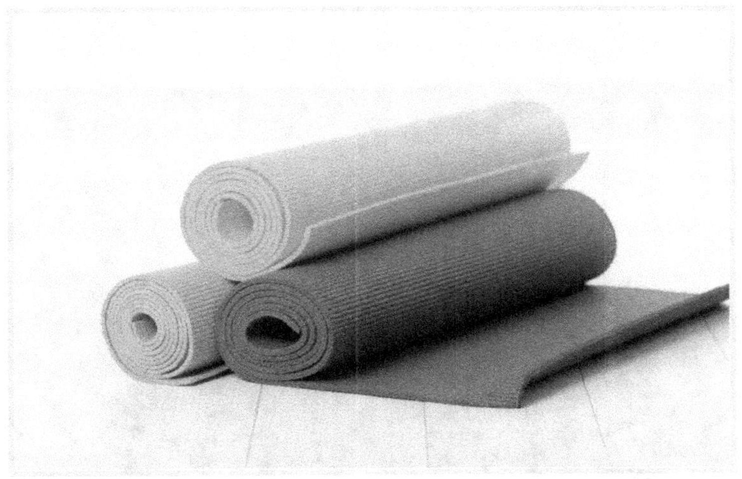

A yoga mat or exercise mat promotes comfort and traction while the wall offers support. When you're on the floor, it guarantees a padded surface for your hands, knees, and back. If you want to avoid slipping, especially during dynamic activities, look for a mat with high grip.

Resistance Bands

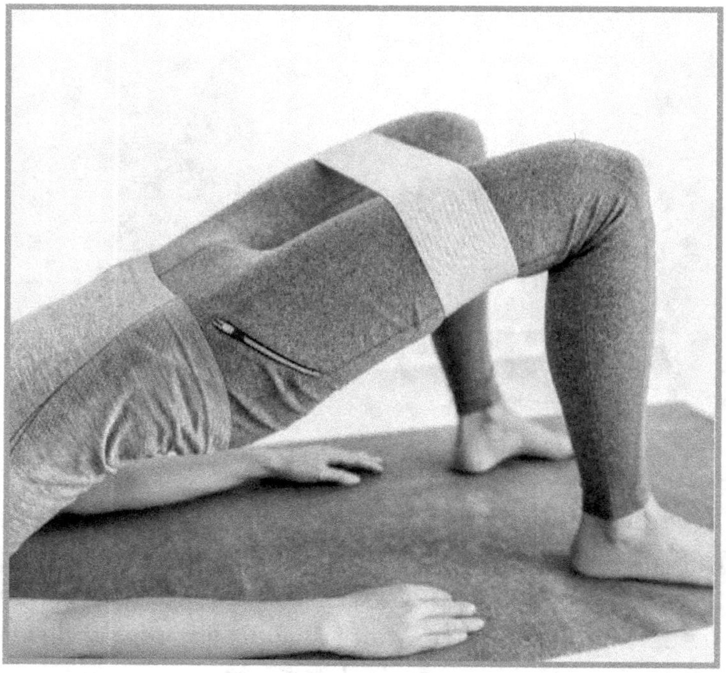

Your Wall Pilates program becomes more challenging and increases muscular engagement when you add resistance. Purchase a set of resistance bands that vary in tension. These bands are adaptable and may be used in a variety of exercises, adding added resistance to routines for the upper and lower bodies.

Stability Ball

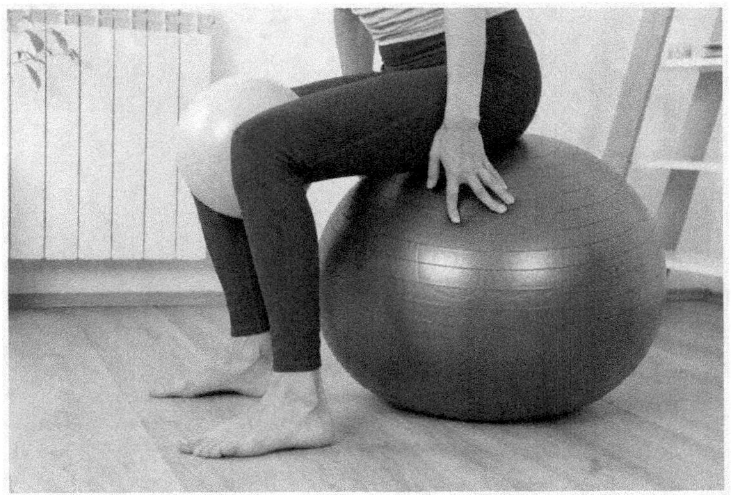

An excellent addition to your Wall Pilates toolkit is a stability ball. It increases the degree of instability, which further works your core muscles. A stability ball adds a humorous aspect to your practice, whether you use it for wall squats or as support during stretching exercises.

Hand Weights or Dumbbells

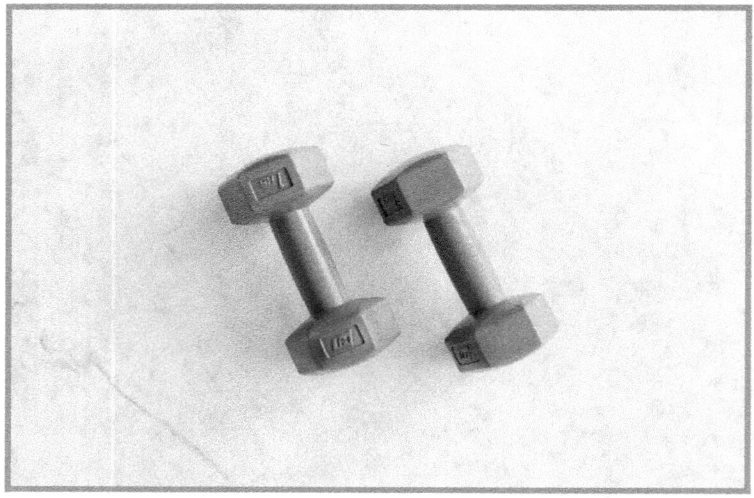

For those looking to intensify their upper body workouts, a pair of hand weights or dumbbells is a fantastic investment. Start with lighter weights and gradually progress as your strength increases. These weights can be used for exercises like wall push-ups, bicep curls, and overhead presses.

Ankle Weights

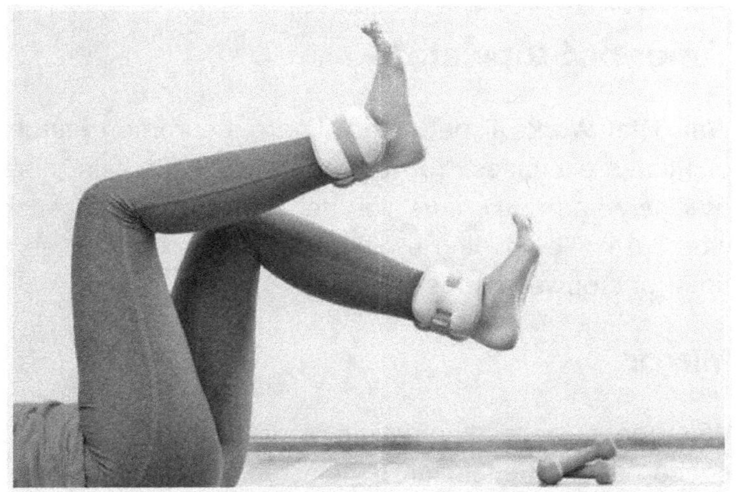

If you want to precisely target your lower body, you might think about using ankle weights. You can add resistance to leg lifts, side leg raises, and other lower body exercises by strapping these around your ankles. They're a delicate yet efficient method of toning and shaping your leg muscles.

Water Bottle and Towel

A water bottle should be kept close by so you can stay hydrated during your Wall Pilates exercise. It's also a good idea to have a towel handy because sweating is an indication of exertion. Especially in activities where you have to lean against the wall, wipe away any sweat to keep your grasp comfortable.

Timer or Stopwatch

Wall That Works Timed intervals are a common feature of Pilates exercises. You can track your intervals more precisely and make sure you get the most out of each workout while keeping a balanced routine if you keep a timer or stopwatch close at hand.

Mirror

While not a necessity, having a mirror in your workout space can be beneficial. It helps you check your form and alignment during exercises. Proper form is crucial in Pilates, and a mirror provides real-time feedback to ensure you're performing each movement correctly.

Comfortable Workout Attire and Shoes

Finally, but just as importantly, dress comfortably for your workouts so that you may move freely. Wall Pilates requires a variety of body positions, so dress comfortably without limiting your range of motion. Choose stable, supportive sports shoes, particularly if your regimen involves standing activities.

Equipped with these fundamental items, you're ready to explore the realm of Wall Pilates. It's important to keep in mind that you should start off slowly and raise the bar for yourself as your flexibility and strength increase. Enjoy the path to a more muscular, stronger version of yourself!

Safety Considerations

Safety must come first in the thrilling world of Wall Pilates to guarantee a joyful and injury-free experience, where every action is a step toward a healthier and stronger you. Let's explore some crucial safety tips that will help you get the most out of your Wall Pilates exercise and maintain your health as the main priority.

1. A proper warm-up

Spend a few minutes warming up your body before beginning the energizing Wall Pilates practice. To improve blood flow to your muscles, try some dynamic stretches or mild aerobic activities. This lessens the possibility of strains or injuries and helps your body get ready for the challenges ahead.

2. Mindful Alignment:

Upon commencing your Wall Pilates journey, be mindful of the alignment of your body. Make sure your shoulders are relaxed, your core is active, and your spine is in a neutral position. In addition to increasing the workouts' efficacy, proper alignment reduces the chance of pain or damage.

3. Gradual Progression:

Although it's great to get proficient at more difficult Wall Pilates exercises, it's important to go slowly. As you gain strength and flexibility, start with basic exercises and work your way up to more difficult ones. Hurrying into complex moves without a firm base puts you at danger for injury and overexertion.

4. Respect Your Limits:

The key to Wall Pilates is to pay close attention to your body. Be mindful of your own boundaries and refrain from overexerting yourself, particularly in the beginning. Since every person's physique is different, it's acceptable to adjust exercises to your comfort level. As your strength increases over time, you can inevitably advance to increasingly strenuous workouts.

5. Quality Over Quantity:

In the realm of Wall Pilates, control and precision are valued more highly than volume of reps. Throughout each exercise, pay close attention to the quality of your movements and maintain good form. This increases the workout's efficacy and lowers the possibility of strain or harm from careless execution.

6. Appropriate Footwear

Make sure your shoes are supportive and comfortable, particularly if your Wall Pilates exercise includes dynamic or standing poses. Good grip and arch support in your shoes can help you stay stable and avoid slipping.

7. Stay Hydrated:

During any strenuous exercise, staying hydrated is essential. To stay properly hydrated, keep a water bottle close by and take little sips throughout your workouts. Maintaining adequate hydration helps to avoid cramps and exhaustion while also supporting muscle function.

8. Safe Wall Distance:

To prevent unintentional impacts, keep a safe distance from the wall during workouts. This is especially crucial while doing exercises that require you to reach or stretch your limbs. A gentle separation guarantees a seamless and injury-free practice.

9. Breath Awareness:

Your Wall Pilates routine will benefit from including attentive breathing. Concentrate on taking deep breaths through your nose and out through your mouth. In addition to improving the passage of oxygen to your muscles, proper breathing eases tension and encourages relaxation.

10. Cool down and stretch:

Never bypass the cooling-off period. Stretching activities will help your body to gradually return to a resting state. This facilitates suppleness and lessens the likelihood of muscular stiffness, making the post-workout recuperation more comfortable.

When you engage in Wall Pilates, make safety your dependable partner. You're protecting your health and improving the overall efficacy and enjoyment of your Wall Pilates experience when you address these factors with awareness. Cheers to a voyage full of health, happiness, and power!

CHAPTER 3: Basic Pilates Principles

Alignment and Posture

Maintaining proper posture can be compared to a hidden superpower that not only makes you appear taller and more self-assured, but it also greatly improves your general health. In the world of Wall Pilates, having perfect alignment and posture is essential to a productive and fruitful workout. Now let's explore the welcoming realm of good alignment and posture, where during your Pilates adventure, your body and the wall become great friends.

Picture your body as a well assembled tower of bricks. From your head to your toes, each block symbolizes a distinct body part. Now, the blocks must be precisely positioned for this skyscraper to stand tall and robust. Let's dissect the fundamentals of posture and alignment so that your tower maintains its stability throughout your Wall Pilates exercises.

1. Head and Neck:

Your head's crown is comparable to your tower's highest point. Keep it raised, as though it's grasping for the heavens. Picture yourself being slowly drawn upward by a cord, making room between your shoulders and ears. This helps to relieve tension on your neck and correct your spine.

2. Shoulders:

Envision your shoulders becoming loose and distancing themselves from your ears. They don't have to bear the weight of the entire globe. This eliminates needless tension and permits a solid base in wall Pilates. It feels like taking a little vacation for your shoulders.

3. Spine:

The main support structure of your tower is your spine. Retain a neutral spine that is neither rounded nor arched. To support your lower back, softly engage your core. Imagine it as a neatly stacked stack of coins, one on the other. This alignment guarantees that the movements you perform during Wall Pilates are efficient and under control.

4. Hips:

The foundation of your tower is your hips. Maintain them squared and level. This firm base makes it possible for muscles to isolate more effectively during Wall Pilates exercises and reduces the needless strain on your lower back. It keeps everything in its proper place, much like a sturdy foundation for a house.

5. Knees:

Bend your knees gently; do not extend them too far. When performing various Pilates exercises against the wall, consider your knees as shock absorbers that are prepared to flex and expand as needed. Additionally, this small bend strengthens your overall stability and guards your joints.

6. Feet:

Spread your feet hip-width apart and firmly plant them on the ground. When you perform Wall Pilates, your feet provide a sense of foundation, much like a tree's roots do. To guarantee a solid contact with the ground, equally divide your weight between both feet. It is the key component for control and balance.

Let's now discuss the enchanted bond that exists between your body and the wall. The wall becomes your quiet ally in wall Pilates, providing support and direction. Feel the comforting, light touch of support as you line up with the wall. It's better to let the wall direct your motions and improve your stability than to forcefully push against it.

During Wall Pilates exercises, observe the way your body moves against the wall. For example, when performing a Wall Sit, your back should be pleasantly pressed up against the wall such that your head and tailbone are in a continuous line. This link guarantees that your muscles are used efficiently, turning the wall into an exercise partner.

It's important to keep in mind that posture and alignment are helpful cues from your body to be conscious, not strict regulations. Accept the organic kinks and motions of your body, enabling it to achieve ideal alignment. You, your body, and the wall are dancing together in a beautiful symphony of flexibility and strength.

Finally, consider posture and alignment to be the unsung heroes of your Wall Pilates journey. They are the beacons of light that increase the efficiency of your exercise regimen by making sure that each movement has a reason and an advantage. Thus, take a stance, align yourself with the wall, and allow the positive energy of proper posture to enhance your Wall Pilates experience. Your body will express gratitude by becoming more flexible, strong, and radiantly well-aware.

Breathing Techniques

Breathing is like learning your body's hidden language in the realm of Wall Pilates, where every breath counts. It's a rhythm, a dance with your inner self that improves the efficiency of your exercise; it's not simply about breathing in and out. Together, we will have a delightful exploration of breathing methods that will improve your Wall Pilates practice.

1. Deep Diaphragmatic Breathing:

To begin, settle into a comfortable position. You can either lie down or sit. Grasp your abdomen with one hand and your chest with the other. Breathe deeply through your nose, causing your abdomen to rise and your diaphragm to dilate. As the air enters your lungs, feel it. Breathe out slowly through your mouth, making sure all of the air is out. Inhaling deeply and diaphragmatically increases oxygen intake, which helps people relax and concentrate.

2. Coordinated Breathing with Movements:

When performing Wall Pilates exercises, synchronize your breathing with your movements. Breathe in during the warm-up and out during the workout. To perform a Wall Squat, for example, inhale as you descend into the squat posture and exhale as you raise yourself back up. This breathing technique creates a smooth workout flow, enhances muscular engagement, and stabilizes your core.

3. Rib Cage Breathing:

Take a comfortable seat with your back straight, and rest your hands on your rib cage's sides. Take a deep breath and spread your ribs laterally. Move the ribs outward with your body. Breathe out slowly, letting your rib cage contract. Breathing from your rib cage increases thoracic mobility, which improves your torso's strength and flexibility.

4. 4-7-8 Breathing Pattern:

This straightforward yet effective breathing pattern entails taking a silent inhale via your nose for four counts, holding it for seven counts, and then loudly expelling through your mouth for eight counts. This method eases tension, soothes the nervous system, and instills a sense of peace in your Wall Pilates exercise.

5. Nose Breathing for Mindfulness:

During Wall Pilates, practice breathing only through your nose. This warms and purifies the air while also fully activating your diaphragm. By promoting awareness, nose breathing helps you to strengthen the mind-body connection and remain in the moment with every activity.

6. Breath Awareness During Stretching:

To get the most out of Wall Pilates' stretching components, pay attention to your breath. Breathe in as you get ready for the stretch and out as you softly enter it. While stretching, mindful breathing reduces stress, increases range of motion, and fosters relaxation.

7. Progressive Relaxation: Breathing techniques:

As you breathe, gradually relax various muscle groups while lying down in a comfortable position. Breathe in deeply, tense a particular muscle group, hold for a little while, and then release the tension by exhaling. Work your way through every muscle group, encouraging general rebirth and relaxation.

Breathing exercises are a vital thread in the beautiful tapestry of Wall Pilates. Accept the beat of your breathing, flow with every motion, and allow the journey of conscious breathing to take your Pilates to new heights. Recall that your breath is the symphony that composes the beauty of your internal journey; it is more than just air.

Core Engagement

The skill of core engagement is one of the fundamentals of Wall Pilates that can greatly improve your practice. Imagine your core as the hub of strength and stability, a powerful area that supports your motions and protects your spine. Let's explore the realm of core engagement and discover the benefits it can offer to your exercise regimen.

Your core is a complicated network of muscles that encircles your torso like a supportive hug; it's not simply about having well-defined abs. Think of it as a strong, organic girdle that supports each movement you perform in a Wall Pilates session.

Let's now discuss technique. Activating your core is like flicking a soft switch that initiates a chain reaction of coordinated muscles. The transverse abdominis, which are the deep abdominal muscles, should be your first emphasis. Just visualizing your belly button moving toward your spine can have a profound effect.

Pay attention to your breathing as you begin your Wall Pilates exercise. A lovely synergy exists in the dance between breath and core engagement. Take a deep breath, letting your rib cage open up, then release it as your core muscles start to tense up. This synchrony gives your practice a meditative character in addition to improving your steadiness.

Keep your center of awareness open during the entire workout. Let your core be your guide when you're practicing wall squats or holding a wall plank. It's about a constant, soft engagement that flows naturally into every movement rather than just crunching or flexing.

You'll observe the positive changes in your posture as you advance. A strong core supports your spine and lowers your chance of strain by acting as a natural corset. It's like putting on a shield for your body, enabling you to confidently do your Pilates exercises.

Recall that the complexity of core engagement is what makes it so beautiful. It's about embracing a mindful relationship with your body, not about pushing or straining. Therefore, allow your core to be your ally and constant companion during each Wall Pilates session as it skillfully and gracefully leads you through a tapestry of moves. Let's explore the amiable force that resides in your core, the unsung hero of your Pilates journey!

CHAPTER 4: Wall Pilates Fundamentals

Wall Sit Basics (Proper Wall Sit Technique)

Now let's get into the correct form for the wall sit, which is a very useful and adaptable workout that greatly improves the strength and endurance of your lower body.

First things first, locate a free wall place for yourself. The ideal surface is one that is level and smooth. Make sure that your feet are hip-width apart while you stand with your back to the wall. At this point, gradually lower yourself until your thighs are parallel to the floor by bending your knees and lowering your torso. It is important to keep your lower back in its natural curve and to keep it comfortably placed against the wall.

Verify the position of your knees; they should be directly above, not extending past, your ankles. This guarantees that your hamstrings and quadriceps are working properly and helps safeguard your knee joints. Try to bring your knees up to a 90-degree angle.

Upon lowering yourself into the wall sit, observe your alignment. From your head to your tailbone, visualize your spine as a straight line. To maintain stability and support your lower back, contract your core muscles.

Let's now discuss weapons. Here, you have a choice! Putting your hands on your hips is a simple method. Lift your arms to shoulder height or extend them straight out in front of you if you want to exercise your upper body a little more. This helps enhance your general balance while also providing an additional challenge.

It's time to discuss that crucial clock. When first starting, try to hold the wall sit for a minimum of thirty seconds. Increase the duration gradually as you gain strength. Recall, quality matters more than quantity. You're doing it correctly if you can feel the burn!

Although breathing is often taken for granted, it is extremely important. Breathe in deeply as you descend into the wall and out gently when you ascend again. Throughout the activity, this regular breathing improves your mind-body connection while also aiding in the oxygenation of your muscles.

Muscles Targeted

Every movement in the realm of Wall Pilates is a symphony of muscle engagement, resulting in a harmonious combination of endurance, flexibility, and strength. Let's examine the subtle differences between the muscles worked in these high-intensity workouts.

1. Core:

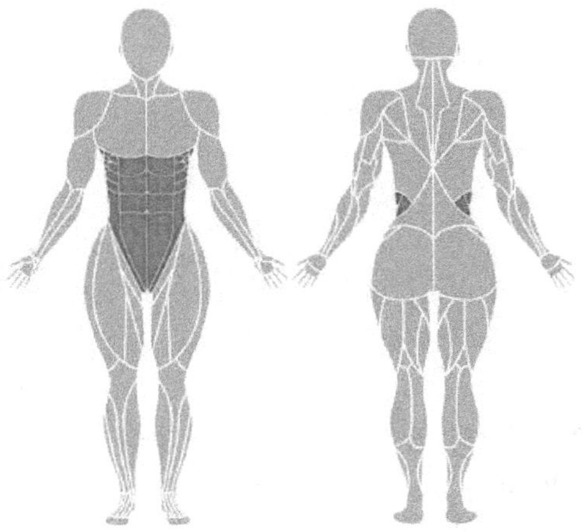

The center of your body and its powerhouse is your core. The deep abdominal muscles, such as the obliques and transverse abdominis, are highlighted in wall Pilates. Not only can a strong and stable core help you tone your stomach, but it can also improve your balance and posture in general.

2. Glutes and Legs:

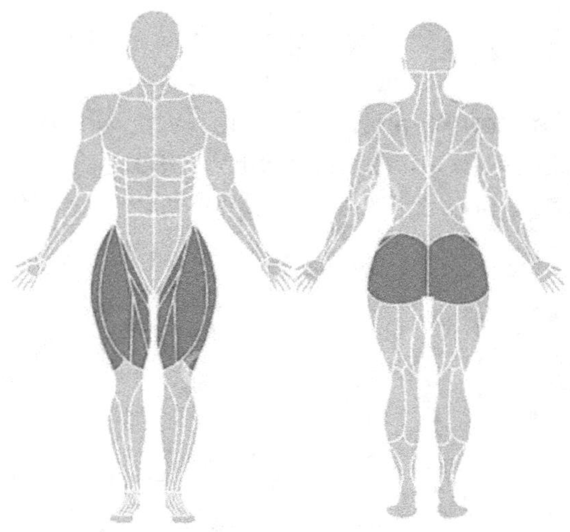

Imagine performing leg circles, wall lunges, and wall squats. These workouts are an ode to your bottom half. Your glutes, hamstrings, and quadriceps become dancing partners, assisting in the development of your strength and grace. The wall exercises' isometric format increases muscle engagement and provides your legs with a demanding yet worthwhile workout.

3. Arms and Shoulders:

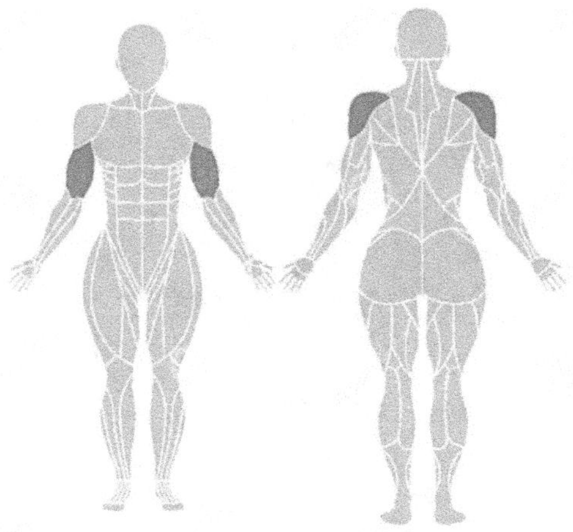

When it comes to Wall Pilates, no muscle is left unworked. Your arms and shoulders will look like sculptural works of art after performing wall push-ups and tricep dips. In addition to toning your biceps and triceps, pushing and pulling against the wall works your shoulder stabilizing muscles, which builds upper body strength and definition.

4. Back Muscles:

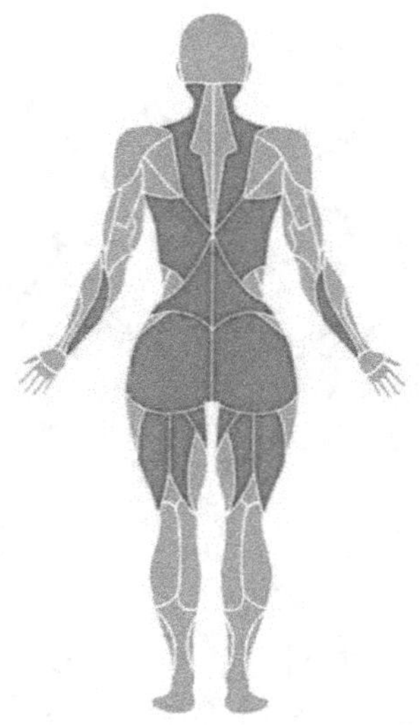

Your back muscles are the unsung heroes of roll-ups and wall bridges. To support your spine and preserve good posture, the erector spinae, lats, and rhomboids cooperate. Wall Pilates not only strengthens but also cares for the sometimes overlooked muscles that support a robust and healthy back.

5. Pelvic Floor:

The Pilates party is open to the subtle but essential pelvic floor muscles. These muscles are engaged by wall exercises, which emphasize stability and controlled motions, improving pelvic floor function. Women can particularly benefit from this, as it can increase their strength and flexibility in this important area.

6. Whole-Body Integration:

The smooth integration of various muscle groups is what makes Wall Pilates genuinely amazing. Every action fits together harmoniously, much like the pieces of a puzzle. Your body becomes a synchronized orchestra that plays a symphony of endurance, flexibility, and strength.

Muscles are not only worked; they are nourished, tested, and appreciated in the world of Wall Pilates. It's more than simply an exercise routine; it's a cordial exchange of words between your body and the wall that crafts a stunning story of health and power.

Common Mistakes and How to Avoid Them

Starting a Wall Pilates program can be a rejuvenating path to health and fitness. However, like with any new undertaking, there will inevitably be some bumps in the road. Don't worry! Let's look at some typical Wall Pilates blunders and, more importantly, how to avoid them with elegance.

1. Poor Wall Sit Posture

The simplicity of a Wall Sit is its charm, but it's simple to overlook proper posture. Excessive forward leaning or disregarding alignment might cause back pain and reduce the workout's effectiveness. Solution: Make sure your knees are bent 90 degrees, your weight is equally distributed on both feet, and your back is flush against the wall.

2. Neglecting Core Engagement

Pilates is all about the core; to ignore it would be to miss the show's main act. When performing planks or leg lifts, neglecting to use your core muscles might cause discomfort and lessen the advantages. Solution: Tighten your abdominal muscles consciously before beginning each activity, and keep them that way throughout.

3. Ignoring Breathing Technique

Although it may seem instinctive, breathing is an art in Pilates. Breathing too slowly or erratically can disrupt your rhythm and impair your performance. Solution: Concentrate on taking slow, deep breaths. For every exercise, take a breath during the preparation stage and release it during the exertion stage.

4. Rushing Through Movements

We may be tempted to speed through workouts in our excitement to see results. This puts form at jeopardy and raises the possibility of injury. Accept the idea that quality matters more than quantity as a solution. Perform each motion with awareness, feeling your muscles contract.

5. Ignoring Flexibility Training

Pilates emphasizes flexibility as much as strength. Reduced range of motion and muscle tension might result from skipping stretches. Solution: Set aside time for stretches. Excellent support for efficient and controlled stretches can be obtained from the wall.

6. Skipping Warming Up

Leaping directly into the wall Pilates without a good warm-up is equivalent to idling a car while it's chilly outside. It's critical to get your body ready for the forthcoming difficulties. Solution: Make a vigorous warm-up a priority to improve blood flow and relax muscles.

7. Relying Too Heavily on the Wall

Although the wall is an excellent instrument for support, depending too much on it can impede your progress. You'll want to develop your strength and balance over time without continual assistance. Solution: As you acquire strength and confidence, gradually lessen your reliance on the wall. Increase the number of standalone workouts you do to challenge yourself.

8. Ignoring Signals of Pain

The adage "no pain, no gain" is not relevant to the Pilates community. Your body uses pain as a warning when something isn't right. Injury is a possibility if you ignore it. Solution: Pay attention to your body. If you feel pain (not the same as the soreness you get from a hard workout), change the exercise or your form.

9. Inconsistency

Steadiness is the foundation of advancement. Your progress toward mastering Wall Pilates may be hampered by missing exercises or inconsistent practice. Solution: Establish a non-negotiable schedule for your regular appointments. The secret to really benefiting from Pilates is consistency.

Keep in mind that every person's Pilates journey is different as you navigate these typical blunders. Accept that you will learn from it, acknowledge your little successes, and never give up on improving your technique. You'll find yourself flying through your Wall Pilates program if you have a thoughtful approach and a positive outlook on your own development.

25-DAY CHALLENGE

Wall Chest Stretch

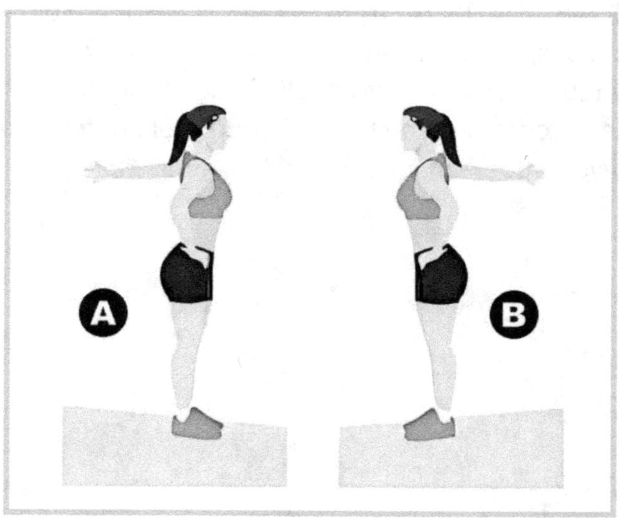

Primary muscles: **Chest**
Equipment: **No equipment**

Instructions

- With the side of your body facing a wall, place your left palm on the wall.
- Slowly rotate your torso to the right, until you feel the stretch in your chest and in your left shoulder.
- Hold for 15 to 30 seconds and repeat on the right side.

Proper Form And Breathing Pattern

Maintain your hand in line with your shoulder and press your palm firmly on the wall while performing the chest stretch. Exhale as you extend the stretch farther, and keep your back straight while you rotate your body and open up your chest.

Exercise Benefits

The wall chest stretch helps to release your shoulder and bicep muscles as well as expand your chest. This stretch also helps to enhance posture, blood circulation, and flexibility.

· **Wall Calf Stretch** ·

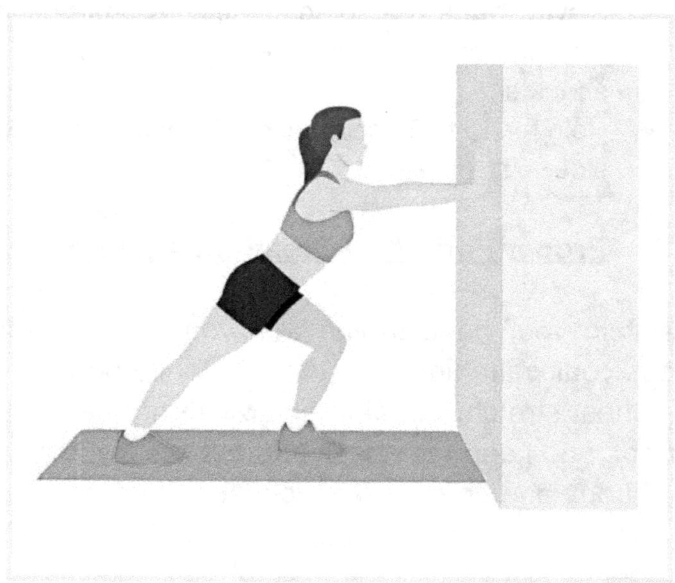

Primary muscles: **Calves**
Equipment: **No equipment**

<u>Instructions</u>

- With your toes pointing forward and your arms outstretched, take a stand gripping a wall.
- With your right foot flat on the ground, extend your right leg back.
- Bend your left knee gradually as you lean forward until your back calf stretches.

- Maintain the stretch, then switch to the left leg.

Proper Form And Breathing Pattern

Keep your feet pointed forward and plant your back heel firmly on the ground. Drop your hips forward and downward while maintaining a straight back knee. Take a deeper breath out and gently extend the stretch without straining.

Exercise Benefits

In reality, the calf muscle is a collection of muscles located on the rear of the lower leg. These muscles support and stabilize your ankles and feet in addition to lifting your heel up to enable forward motion. You may significantly lessen stress and increase stability and flexibility by stretching your calves.

· Leg up the wall stretch ·

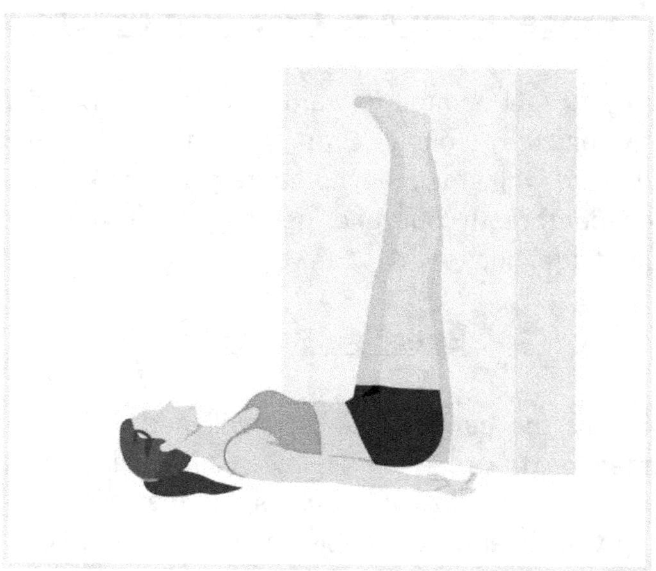

Primary muscles: **Quadriceps, Hamstrings & Calves**
Equipment: **No equipment**

<u>Instructions</u>

- As comfortable as possible, place your sitting bones against the wall while lying on your back.
- Raise your legs up the wall until your backs are completely flat on it.
- Hold this position for ten to fifteen minutes.

<u>Exercise Benefits</u>

An inversion stance that can assist counteract gravity's effects on the body as a whole is legs up the wall. This posture stimulates digestion, balances blood pressure, and aids in the removal of toxins and fluids from the body. When paired with focused breathing. Your body will begin to recover and restore itself as a result, lowering your levels of tension and anxiety.

· Wall Hip Flexor ·

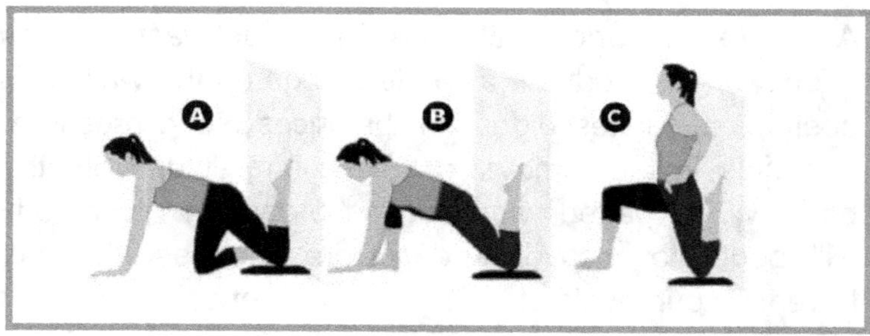

Primary muscles: **Iliopsoas and rectus femoris**
Equipment: **No equipment**

Instructions

- Keep the knee support near the wall.
- As a first step, get into a kneeling position.
- Slide one of the knees onto the pad which is close to the edge of the wall as shown in figure A
- As demonstrated in picture B, the Low Lunge posture now extends one knee forward at a right angle while maintaining the other knee near the wall. Achieve ankle plantar flexion, or the position where the toes of the foot hitting the wall point upward. Maintain this posture for a few seconds.

- As you extend your hip flexors, take a position where your hands are on your knees and raise your torso with them.
- Continue forcing your torso erect until your glutes come into contact with the floor, landing in the high lunge position depicted in figure C. Hold this position for 20 seconds.
- Maintain a straight torso, hips, and knees at all times, and contract your glutes.

Exercise Benefits

The rectus femoris and iliopsoas are two of the hip flexor muscles that are the main focus of wall hip flexor workouts. These muscles are essential for hip flexion, which enables you to bend at the waist or raise your knees toward your chest. Walking, running, and cycling are just a few of the activities that require strong hip flexors. You may specifically work on strengthening and extending these muscles using wall hip flexor exercises, which can lead to increased flexibility, less tightness, and greater hip function overall.

· Wall Calf Raising ·

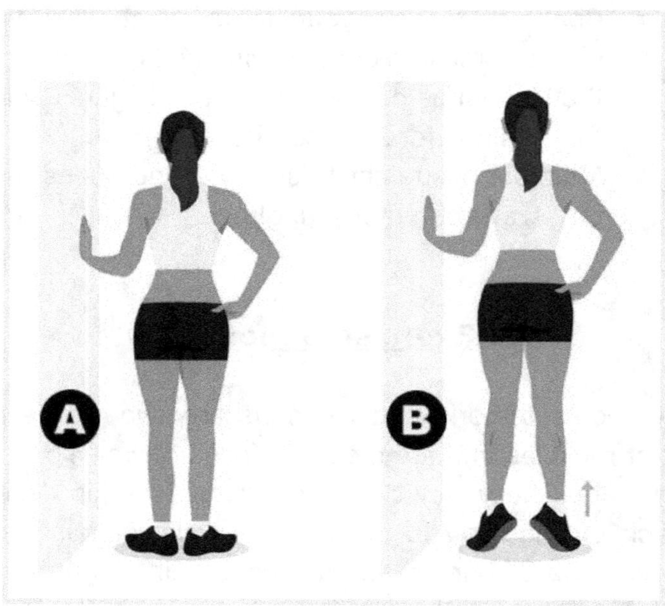

Primary Muscle: **Calf**
Equipment: **No Equipment**

<u>Instructions</u>

- Stand up straight with both feet flat on the floor, slightly apart. Place your hands on the wall or hold onto a sturdy chair, railing, counter, or table.

- Raise both heels so you're standing on the balls of your feet. Don't lock your knees or arch your back. Hold for 5 seconds. Then slowly lower your heels back down to the floor.

- Repeat

Exercise Benefits

Exercises that raise the leg muscles have the advantage of strengthening and toning the calves' muscles. This helps to increase functional performance in motions like walking, running, and jumping as well as increased ankle stability. Additionally, by encouraging greater muscle control and endurance, calf raises can help prevent lower limb injuries. By including calf raises on a regular basis, you may strengthen your lower body generally and develop stronger, more resilient lower leg muscles.

Lateral Leg Swing

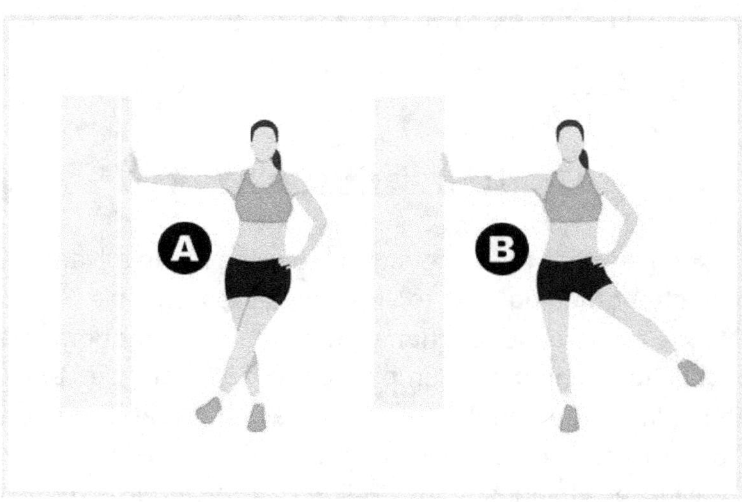

Primary muscles: **Hips**
Equipment: **No equipment**

Instructions

- Stand tall and hold onto a wall.
- Shift your weight to the right leg and swing your left leg to the left and then across your body to the right.
- Repeat the movement with the right leg until the set is complete.

Proper Form And Breathing Pattern

Keep your core tight and your torso still. Use your muscles, not your momentum, to move your legs slowly and deliberately. Breathe slowly, and attempt to get your leg closer to its maximum range of motion with each leg swing.

Exercise Benefits

By extending your hip range of motion, lateral leg swings get your muscles, tendons, and joints ready for further physical exertion. Dynamic stretches help us stay injury-free and increase our performance throughout exercise.

Double V Wall Stretch

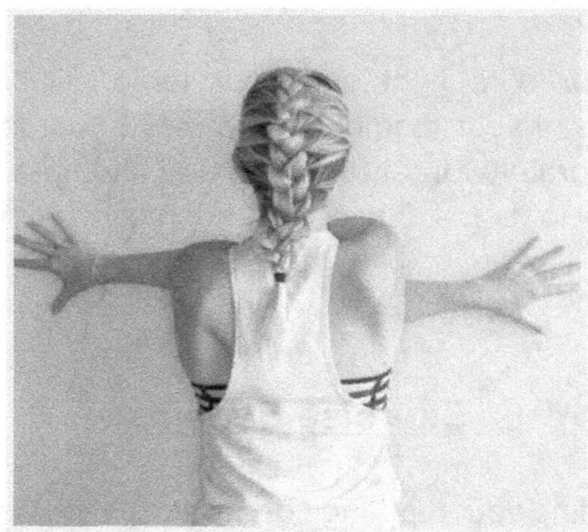

Primary muscles: **Hips**
Equipment: **No equipment**

Instructions

- Position yourself about arm's length away from a wall. Stand tall with your feet shoulder-width apart.
- Extend your arms straight in front of you and place your palms on the wall at shoulder height. Your fingers should be pointing upward.
- Keeping your hands in the same spot, slowly walk them down the wall. Bring your chest down to the floor.

- As you walk your hands down, your body will naturally form a V shape. Keep your arms straight and your head between your shoulders.
- Your upper back, chest, and shoulders should all feel slightly stretched. You can deepen the stretch by walking your hands down further if you're more flexible.
- While holding the extended posture for 20 to 30 seconds, take deep breaths. Concentrate on unwinding into the stretch and experiencing the release of tension.

Exercise Benefits

An effective exercise for relieving tension in the shoulders, neck, and upper back is the double v wall stretch. Your arms and torso should form a V against the wall to promote a mild stretch that can reduce stiffness and increase flexibility in these areas. This stretch is very useful for people who are suffering from tight muscles or pain from sitting at a desk. Better posture and a greater sense of upper body relaxation can be achieved with regular practice.

Wall DownDog

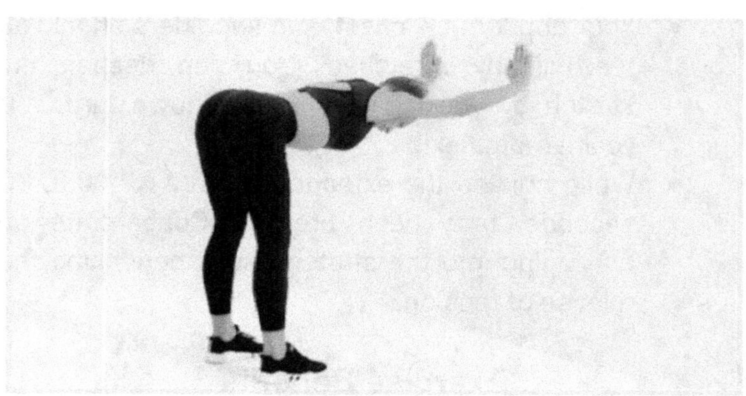

Primary muscles: **Pectoral Muscles & Lats**
Equipment: **No equipment**

Instructions

- Standing a few feet away with your feet hip-width apart. Place your hands on the wall at shoulder height, fingers spread, creating a comfortable and stable base.
- Hinge at your hips, maintaining a straight line from your wrists to your tailbone. Allow your chest to move toward the wall while extending your legs, creating an inverted V shape with your body.
- Make sure your legs and spine are in proper alignment, and firmly plant your heels on the

ground. throughout the length of your spine and throughout your hamstrings and calves, feel the mild stretch.

Exercise Benefits

One useful exercise for both strengthening and stretching different muscle areas is the wall downward dog. This pose helps extend the calves, hamstrings, and spine. Place your hands on the floor and your feet against the wall. It improves stability and balance by activating the shoulders and core. This is an especially good exercise for increasing general flexibility, releasing back tightness, and promoting relaxation. Including the Wall Downward Dog in your practice can help your body become more flexible and agile.

LEVEL 2 ★★

· Wall Push Ups ·

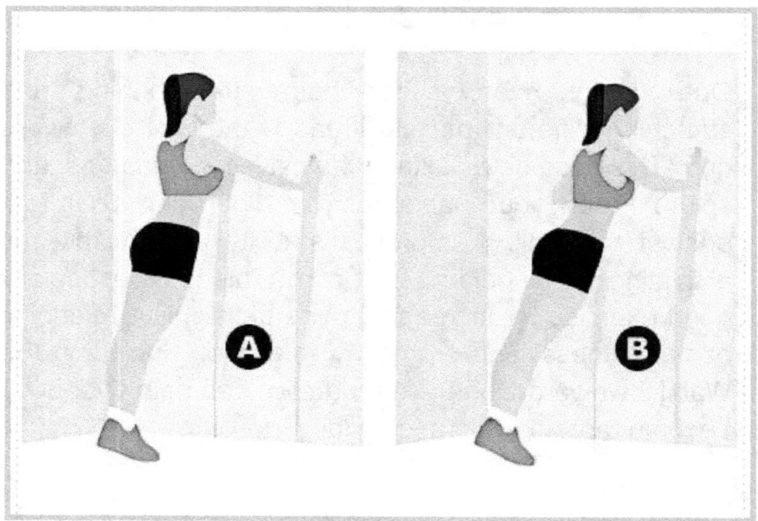

Primary muscles: **Chest & Triceps**
Equipment: **No equipment**

Instructions

- Stand facing a wall, about arm's length away.
- Place your hands on the wall at shoulder height, slightly wider than shoulder-width apart.
- Maintain a straight body from head to heels.
- Make use of your core muscles to keep yourself stable.

- Bend your elbows, lowering your chest toward the wall.
- Inhale as you lower your body.
- Exhale and push through your palms to straighten your arms.
- Focus on using your chest and triceps to push back.

Exercise Benefits

There are several advantages to wall push-ups, including stronger upper limbs, more stable cores, and more flexibility in the shoulders. This adaptable workout is easy on the joints, so people of all fitness levels may do it. Wall push-ups are a great complement to any well-rounded fitness program because they improve posture and increase total upper body training.

· Side Plank ·

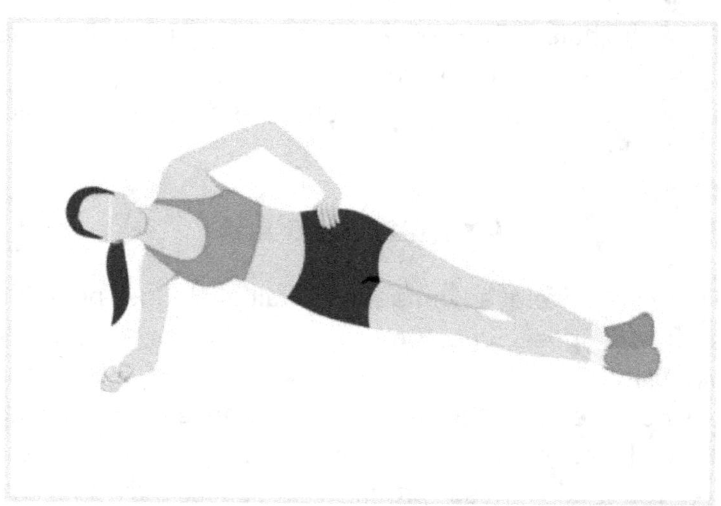

Primary muscles: **Core**
Equipment: **No equipment**

Instructions

- Extend your body fully while lying on your side.
- Elevate your body off the ground and distribute your weight evenly between your forearm and your foot's side.
- Hold the position for as long as you can, keeping your body in a straight line.
- Switch sides and carry on.

Exercise Benefits

One of the main advantages of the Side Plank exercise is that it works and strengthens the lateral muscles of the core, especially the obliques. This lateral stability improves general core strength, which in turn promotes better posture and balance, in addition to helping to sculpt the waist. The Side Plank also works the knees, hips, and shoulders, giving the full body a thorough exercise. By performing this exercise regularly, you can develop a stronger core, more endurance, and better lateral strength.

· Wall Sit ·

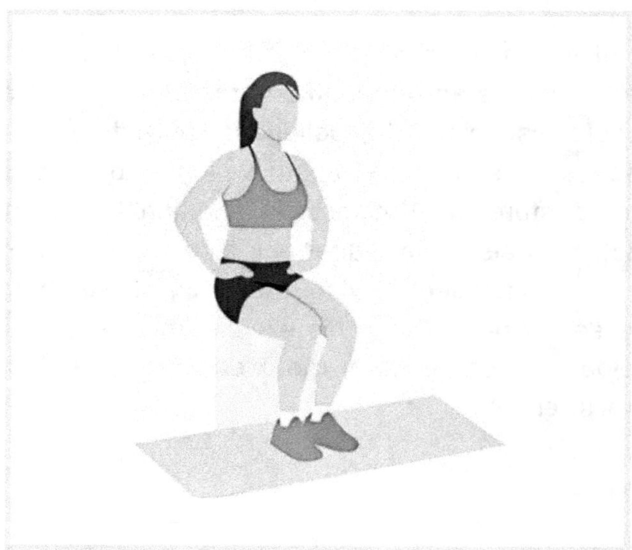

Primary muscles: **Thighs**
Equipment: **No equipment**

Instructions

- With your back against a wall and your thighs parallel to the floor, begin in the squat posture.
- For as long as you can, maintain this posture.

Exercise Benefits

Wall sits have the added benefit of exercising multiple muscle groups at once. This works especially well for strengthening the quadriceps, hamstrings, and glutes. Because the exercise is isometric, it works the core muscles, which improves general lower body strength and stability. Including wall sits in your regimen helps you maintain better posture, tone your legs, and build a stronger foundation for everyday tasks.

Dumbbell Side Bend

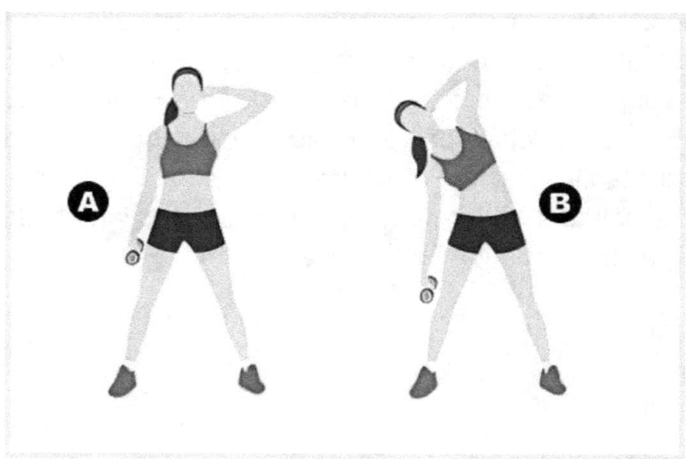

Primary muscles: **Obliques**
Equipment: **Dumbbell**

Instructions

- Place your feet shoulder-width apart and take a tall stance. With your left hand behind your head, hold a dumbbell in your right hand with the palm facing your hip.

- Pause and slant to your right side as far as is comfortable.

- Continue doing this for the whole set, then switch sides.

Exercise Benefits

The obliques, or the muscles on the sides of your belly, are the main target of the dynamic exercise known as the dumbbell side bend. This exercise encourages lateral flexion, which tones and strengthens the muscles surrounding your waist. Beyond appearance, the workout helps with better posture and core stability. You may improve your general functional strength and assist activities that require twisting or bending by including Dumbbell Side Bends into your program.

· Wall Squat ·

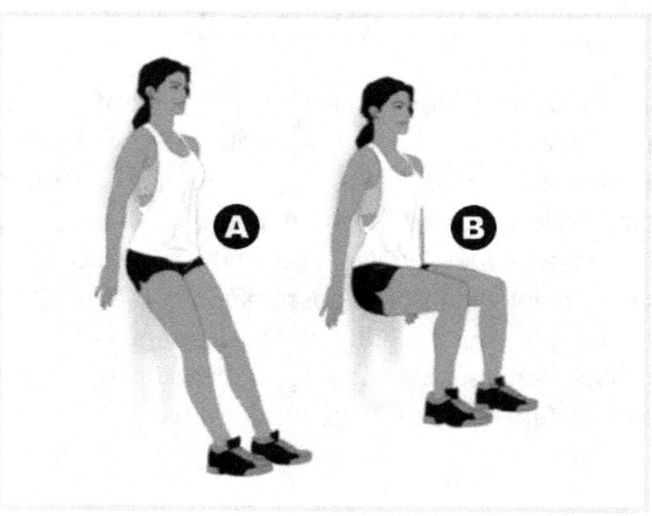

Primary muscles: **Quadriceps, Hamstrings, Gluteal muscles (Buttocks).**
Equipment: **No Equipment.**

Instructions

- Stand so that your back is against the wall, feet placed about 1-2 feet from the wall.

- Bend the knees as you move into a squat until your knees are at a 90 degree angle – your back should stay pressed against the wall at all times.

- After 15 seconds, maintain this posture and stand back up to resume. After 30 seconds of rest, continue the process once more.

Exercise Benefits

There are many advantages to wall squats, including stronger lower body muscles, higher muscle tone in the quadriceps, hamstrings, and glutes, and improved stability. With your knees bent and your back against the wall, this exercise is a great method to improve your squatting form and increase your endurance. In addition, wall squats are less taxing on the knees than regular squats, which makes them a good choice for people who have knee problems. Wall squats are a great way to strengthen your lower body and improve your overall functional fitness.

Single-Leg Knee Crunch

This isn't just a crunch for your abs. You may strengthen your core stability and protect your spine even when your limbs are moving by concentrating on one leg at a time and pressing the other foot against the wall.

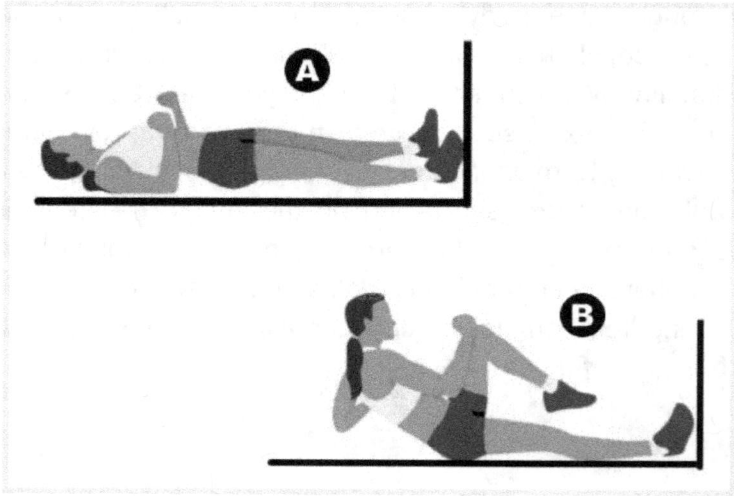

Primary Muscles: **Core or Abs, Obliques & Quadriceps**
Equipment: **No Equipment.**

Instructions

- Place yourself on your back and take a seat approximately a foot away from a wall. Put your legs in a tabletop position by placing your feet flat on the wall.

- Stretch your left leg diagonally till your toes are just slightly above the wall. To activate your core, extend your arms upward and firmly plant your lower back on the ground. This is where you are supposed to start.
- Draw your left knee in toward your chest while simultaneously curling your shoulders off the floor. Then, draw your arms toward the wall so they're next to your hips.
- Slowly release the crunch, returning to the starting position. That's one rep.

Exercise Benefits

The exercise known as the Single-Leg Knee Crunch targets the abdominal muscles with great intensity. This exercise requires balance and core strength, and it calls for a controlled contraction as you bring one leg up to your chest. This exercise helps to improve core stability and can help to tone and sculpt the stomach by isolating and challenging the abdominal region. Including the Single-Leg Knee Crunch in your exercise regimen can help you develop stronger core muscles and a more toned and robust midsection.

• **Wall Bridge** •

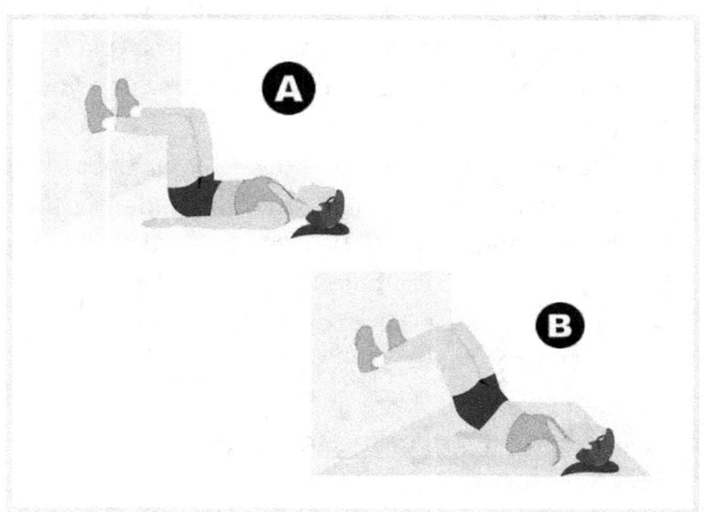

Primary muscles: **Glutes**
Equipment: **No equipment**

<u>Instructions</u>

- Lie on your back with your arms by your sides,
  plant the soles of your feet on a wall, with your
  feet hip-width apart, knees bent, legs at a
  90-degree angle, and your thighs perpendicular
  to the floor.

- Lift your hips as high as you can while tightening your glutes.

- Once the set is finished, go back to the beginning and repeat.

Exercise Benefits

The Wall Bridge exercise is very beneficial since it targets and strengthens the muscles in the lower back, hamstrings, glutes, and core. By placing your back against the wall and raising your hips toward the ceiling, you can improve your posture and pelvic stability with this exercise. Wall Bridge is a useful addition for anyone looking for a comprehensive approach to strength and stability because it helps you develop a more flexible and resilient lower body.

• Thread the Needles •

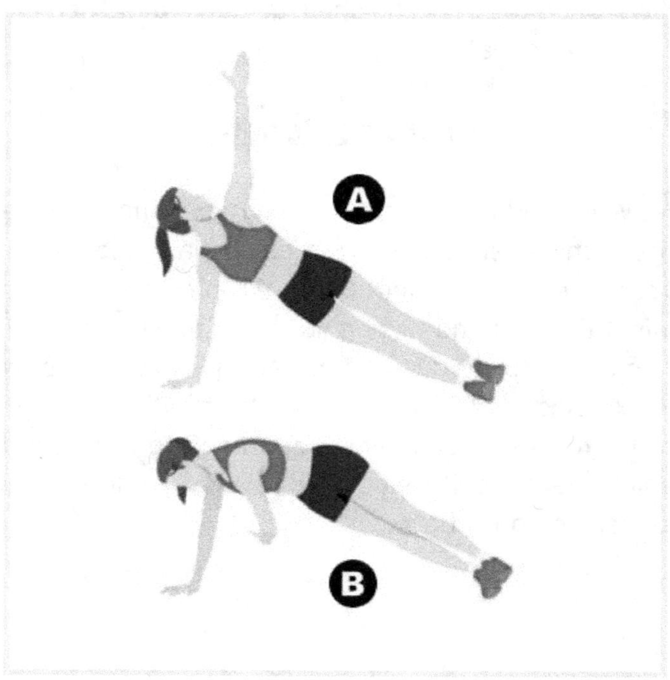

Primary Muscle Groups: **Side Shoulders, Front Shoulders, Rear Shoulders, Lats (back)**
Equipment: **No Equipment**

Instructions

- Start on your side on the floor with your elbow directly underneath your shoulder and feet and knees stacked.

- Lift your hips up into a side plank with your free arm up toward the ceiling.

- Take your free arm and thread it through the open space underneath you while you rotate your shoulders and hips toward the floor.

Exercise Benefits

The Thread the Needle exercise offers a notable benefit by targeting the muscles of the shoulders, upper back, and spine. This movement enhances flexibility and mobility in these areas while also promoting relaxation. The gentle rotation involved in threading the needle helps release tension, making it a valuable exercise for those seeking relief from stiffness or discomfort in the upper body. Regular incorporation of this exercise into your routine can contribute to improved posture and a greater sense of overall upper body well-being.

• **Wall Crunch** •

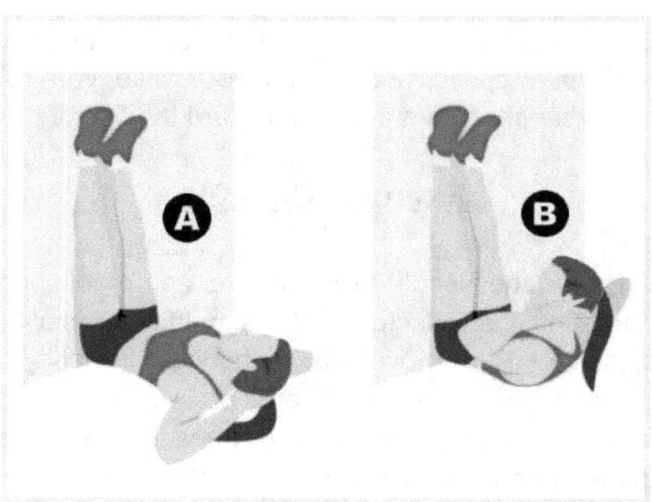

Primary muscles: **Abs**
Equipment: **No equipment**

<u>Instructions</u>

- Lie on your back with your buttocks close to and facing the wall.
- Extend your legs straight up, placing the soles of your feet against the wall.
- Your body should form an L-shape, with your legs perpendicular to the floor.

- Put your hands behind your head and support your neck with your fingers. Do not pull on your head.
- Activate your abdominal muscles by drawing your belly button towards your spine. This engages your core for the upcoming movement.
- Make sure your ribs are close to your hips as you lift your head and shoulders off the ground.

- Inhale as you slowly lower your head and shoulders back to the starting position.

<u>Exercise Benefits</u>

Incorporating the support of a wall into the Wall Crunch exercise makes it a fun and effective way to work your abs. This move works the rectus abdominis and obliques, which are also known as the "six-pack" muscles. By using the wall as a support, the exercise encourages a controlled and focused tightening of the core, which helps build strength and tone. The Wall Crunch also helps you breathe more mindfully, which improves the link between your mind and body during your abdominal workout. Adding this exercise to your routine can help you get stronger in your core and keep your abs healthy in general.

• **Wall Glute Bridge** •

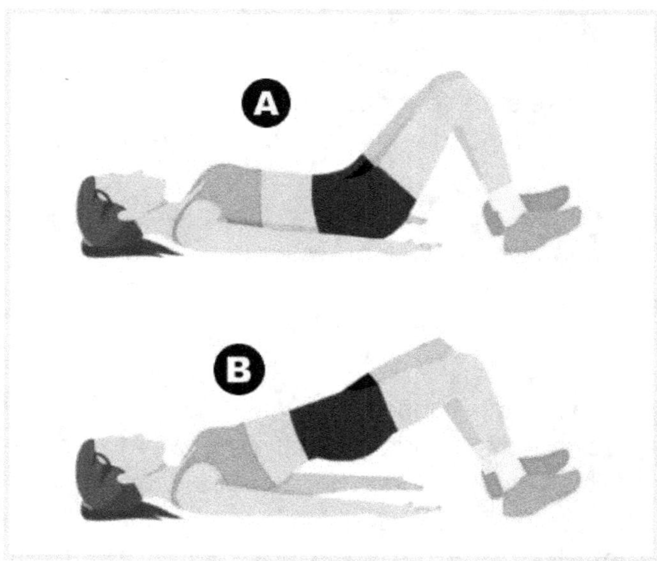

Primary muscles: **Glutes**
Equipment: No equipment

<u>Instructions</u>

- Tighten your abdominal and buttock muscles by pushing your low back into the ground.

- Raise your hips to create a straight line from your knees to your shoulders.

- Squeeze your core and pull your belly button back toward your spine.

- Hold for 20 to 30 seconds.

- Lower the hips to return to the starting position.

Exercise Benefits

Performing Glute Bridges is very helpful because it targets and strengthens the muscles in your buttocks, especially the gluteus maximus. This exercise promotes improved hip stability, enhances lower back support, and adds to better overall posture. Additionally, Glute Bridges work the core muscles, which makes the abs stronger and improves overall lower body health. Adding Glute Bridges to your workout routine on a regular basis can help you perform better in sports, feel less pain in your lower back, and get a more toned and strong back.

• **Wall Split Squat** •

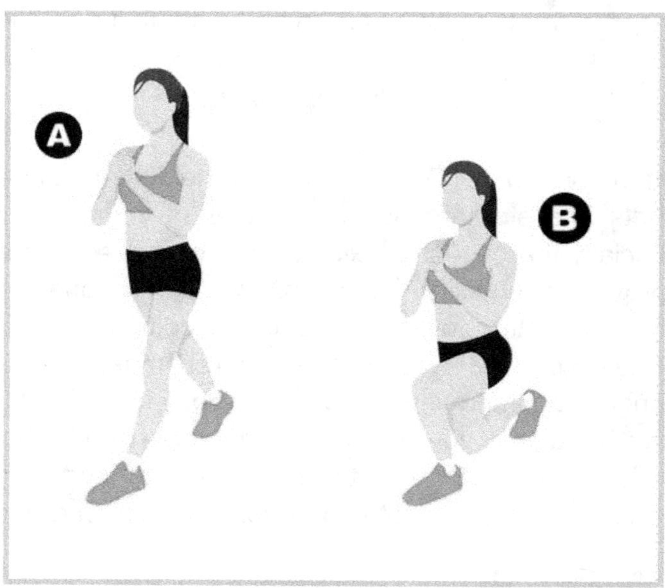

Primary muscles: **Quads**
Equipment: **No equipment**

<u>Instructions</u>

- Stand with feet hip-width apart.
- Take a step forward with one foot, creating a staggered stance.
- Lower your body so that your knees are bent.

- Maintain a straight front knee above the ankle.
- Make sure your rear knee is slightly elevated above the floor.
- Retain your torso upright.
- Use your core to maintain stability.
- Maintain a balanced weight distribution between your two legs.
- Push through your front heel to return to the starting position.
- Complete the desired repetitions on one leg before switching.

Exercise Benefits

Including split squats in your exercise regimen has significant advantages. This dynamic workout develops lower body strength and stability by working the quadriceps, hamstrings, and glutes, among other muscle groups. Split squats also work the core, which improves balance and coordination. This compound action is an essential part of a well-rounded fitness program since it improves joint flexibility in addition to muscular tone.

• **Plank Walk Up** •

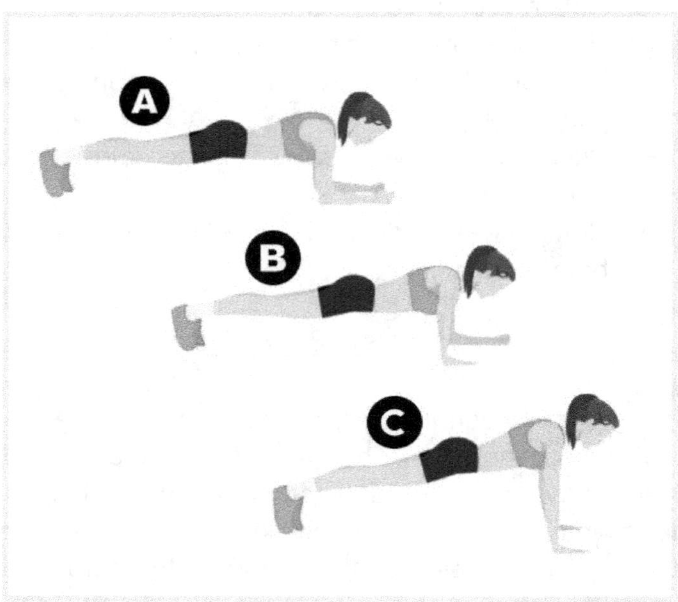

Primary muscles: **Core, abdominis & obliques**
Equipment: **No equipment**

Instructions

- Get into plank position, forearms on the floor, elbows under your shoulders, legs extended behind you.
- Place your right hand flat on the floor

- Then your left, straightening your arms to pushup position
- Return to start by lowering onto your right, then left, forearms. Repeat, leading with your left hand (so you don't burn out arm more than the other); alternate. Perform 3 sets of 8-12 each side.

Exercise Benefits

Engaging in the Plank Walk-Up exercise offers a range of benefits, including enhanced core strength, improved shoulder stability, and increased endurance. This dynamic movement challenges multiple muscle groups simultaneously, promoting better overall functional fitness. The plank walk-up also targets the arms and chest, contributing to upper body toning. Incorporating this exercise into your routine can foster greater body awareness, coordination, and an intensified core engagement, making it a valuable addition to your fitness regimen.

• Wall Sit Leg Lifts •

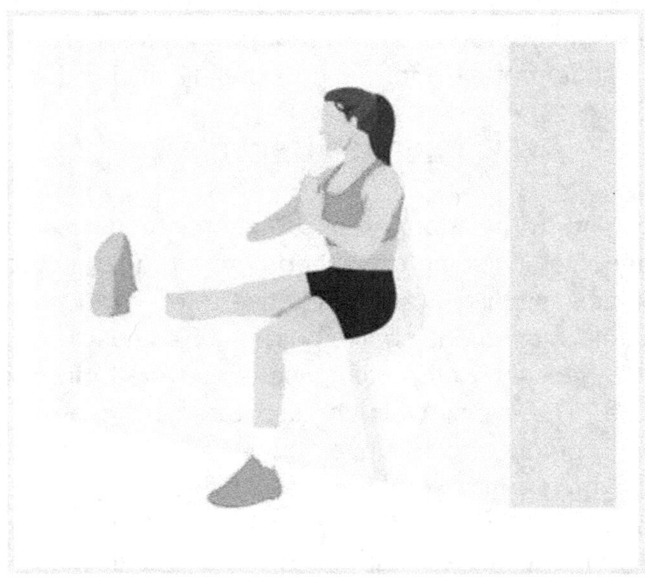

Primary muscles: **Quadriceps, hamstrings, glutes, and calves**
Equipment: **No equipment**

<u>Instructions</u>

- Put your back to a wall while standing.
- Lower your body into a wall sit position, ensuring your back is flat against the wall, and your knees are bent at a 90-degree angle.

- Pull your belly button in the direction of your spine to engage your core muscles.
- Lift one leg off the ground while maintaining the wall sit position.
- Extend your lifted leg forward, keeping it straight and parallel to the ground.
- Maintain the extended position briefly, focusing on balance and control.
- Return the raised leg to its starting position gradually.
- On the opposite leg, repeat the same procedure.

Exercise Benefits

Combining the dynamic movement of leg lifts with the isometric strength of a wall sit provides a twofold benefit when performing wall sit leg lifts. In addition to targeting and strengthening the quadriceps, hamstrings, and glutes during the wall sit, this exercise also works the lower abdominal muscles and hip flexors as you elevate your legs. Combining these components results in a thorough lower body workout that enhances general lower body function, toning, and muscle endurance.

• Ultimate Pike •

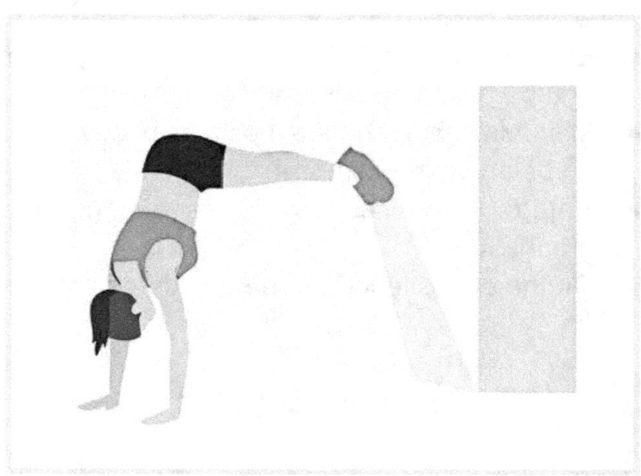

Primary muscles: **Arms, chest, back & core**
Equipment: No equipment

Instructions

- Start by placing your feet hip-width apart and facing the wall.
- Place your hands on the floor, shoulder-width apart, and walk your feet up the wall, coming into an inverted V position. Your body should form an angle with the wall.
- Make sure your hips are piled over your shoulders, your shoulders should be squarely

above your wrists, and your arms should be straight.

- Engage your core muscles and lift your hips toward the ceiling, bringing your body into a pike position. Your legs should be straight, and your heels may touch the wall.
- With a strong shoulder and engaged core, try to form a straight line from your wrists to your hips.
- Hold the pike position for a moment, focusing on stability and maintaining the proper form.
- Slowly lower your hips back down to the starting inverted V position, maintaining control.

Exercise Benefits

The Wall Ultimate Pike exercise targets several muscle groups at once, providing a complete workout. This dynamic exercise strengthens, stabilizes, and stretches the legs, shoulders, and core. Including the Wall Ultimate Pike in your exercise regimen will help you develop better posture, stronger abs, and more general body strength. This exercise is a great complement to a well-rounded fitness program because it works several muscle groups in a coordinated way.

• Bicycle Crunch •

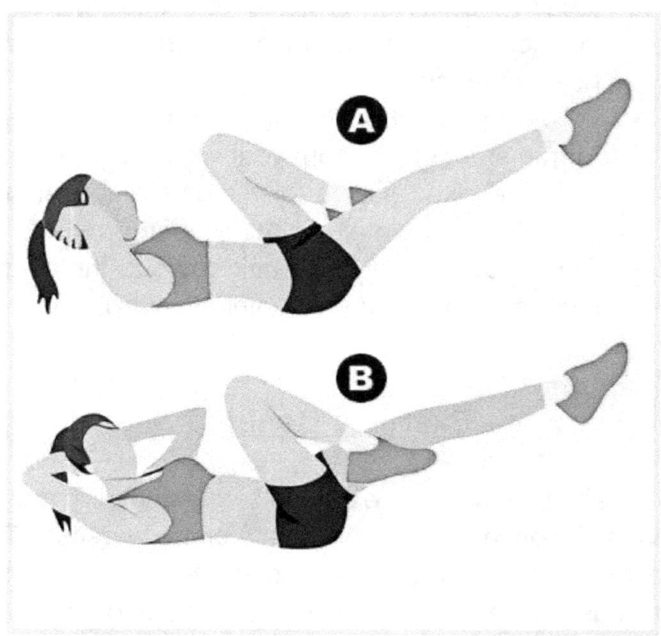

Primary muscles: **Core**
Equipment: No equipment

Instructions

- With your fingers interlocked, support your head gently with your hands while lying on your back.
- Lift your legs off the ground, forming a 90-degree angle at your hips and knees.

- Start by straightening your right leg and bringing your right elbow and left knee closer to one another.
- Simultaneously, twist your torso to bring your left elbow towards your right knee.
- Reverse the motion, straightening your right leg and bringing your left elbow towards your right knee.
- Keep pedaling in this alternate manner while using your core muscles.
- Focus on executing the exercise with controlled, fluid movements rather than speed.
- Keep your lower back pressed into the floor to maximize abdominal engagement and minimize strain.

Exercise Benefits

A dynamic workout that works the obliques and hip flexors in addition to the abdominal muscles is offered by bicycle crunches. This exercise improves coordination and balance while also strengthening and stabilizing the core. The twisting motion is beneficial for toning the entire torso and for shaping the waist. Including bicycle crunches in your regimen can help you develop a strong core, which is important for a variety of everyday tasks and motions. It will also increase your abdominal strength.

• Spiderman Plank •

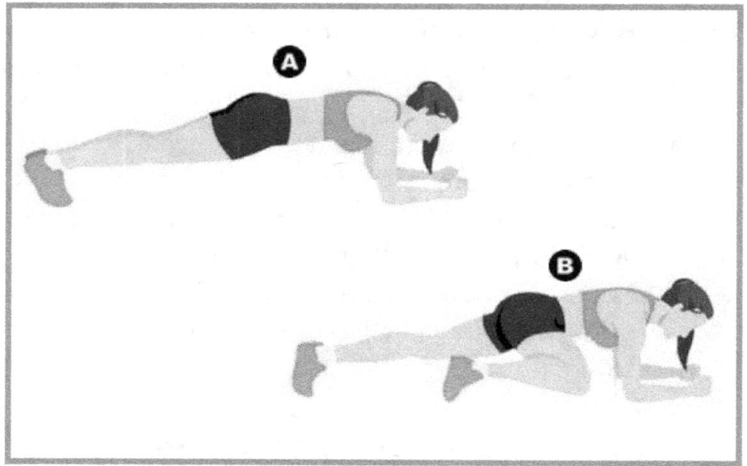

Primary muscles: **Core**
Equipment: **No equipment**

<u>Instructions</u>

- Start in the standard plank posture, with your body in a straight line from head to heels, your arms straight, and your hands directly beneath your shoulders. Make use of your core muscles.

- With the intention of touching or coming as close as you can, raise your right foot off the ground and bring your right knee up to your right elbow.

Avoid lifting your hips too high and maintain a level hip position.

- Take a moment to pause in the Spiderman pose, making sure your knee is up to your elbow. As you maintain the position, notice the contraction in your lower abdomen and obliques.

- Slowly return your right leg to the starting plank position, maintaining control and keeping your body in a straight line.

- Repeat the same sequence with your left leg

Exercise Benefits

A dynamic exercise that provides a special combination of hip flexor activation and core engagement is the Spiderman Plank. This exercise tests stability and mobility while also toning the abdominal muscles. The Spiderman Plank, with its knee-to-elbow motion, targets the obliques and builds a stronger, more resilient midsection. The exercise also improves total control and awareness of the body, which helps with coordination. By incorporating the Spiderman Plank into your routine on a regular basis, you may improve your posture, strengthen your core, and feel more stable when performing other types of physical activity.

• Russian Twists •

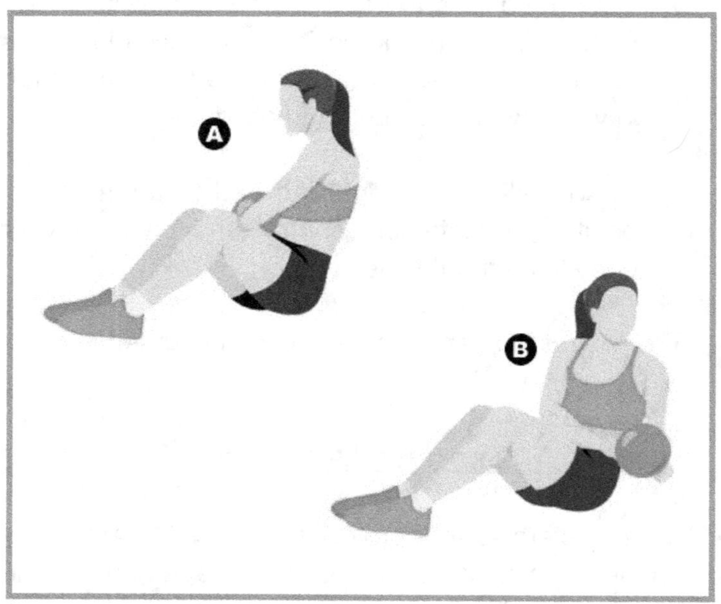

Primary muscles: **Core**
Equipment: **Stability Ball**

<u>Instructions</u>

- Sit on the floor with your knees bent and your feet flat on the floor to start. Maintaining a straight back, slant a little backward and contract your abdominal muscles.

- Hold your hands together in front of you, or clasp them, and lift your feet off the ground, balancing on your sit bones. This creates a V-shape with your torso and thighs.
- Rotate your torso to one side, bringing your hands or clasped hands towards the floor beside your hip. Keep your gaze following your hands to ensure a complete twist.
- Feel the contraction in your obliques as you hold the twisted position for a brief period of time. Make sure you stay balanced on your sit bones the entire time, and keep your feet raised.
- Repeat the motion by slowly circling back to the middle and then twisting to the other side. Maintain a controlled rotation pattern between the sides, paying attention to your torso's rotation and activating your core the entire time.

Exercise Benefits

Incorporating Russian Twists into your exercise regimen enhances torso stability by strengthening your core and obliques. This workout works a variety of muscle groups, improving your overall strength in your abdomen and helping you to maintain better posture. Russian Twists' rotational element contributes to increased spinal flexibility and mobility, which supports a more agile and functional body. Adding Russian Twists on a regular basis can be beneficial for people who want to have a strong, well-rounded core and tone their stomach.

How to maintain your motivation to exercise

Starting a Wall Pilates program is a great way to dedicate yourself to your health, but let's face it: staying motivated may be a little difficult. Everyone has experienced the sense of having their initial excitement gradually fade. But do not panic! Here are some helpful hints to maintain the intensity of your Wall Pilates practice:

First of all, diversity adds flavor to life—and the same goes for your exercise regimen! Don't be afraid to experiment. Add new exercises to your arsenal for Wall Pilates, try out different combinations, and play around with different sequences. This prevents monotony from setting in by keeping things exciting and presenting your body with new challenges.

Having realistic goals changes everything. Divide your goals into more manageable, achievable targets. Enjoy each little victory you achieve along the way, whether it's learning a new leg lift technique or managing to hold a Wall Plank for an additional ten seconds. Acknowledging your progress gives you more self-assurance and motivates you to keep going. Think about joining a community or finding a Wall Pilates partner. Creating a support network with others through sharing your struggles, triumphs, and experiences may really make a big difference. Having a companion on the journey, be it a local acquaintance or a virtual group, enhances the experience and provides an additional level of accountability.

Your ally in the quest for motivation may be music. Make a playlist with the songs that you love and that make you feel excited and motivated. You may turn your workout from a chore into a dance party (yes, I just used the word "D" with the proper music). Bring some fun into your routine by letting the beat dictate how you move.

Recall that it's natural to experience low motivation days. When it happens, try not to be too hard on yourself. Your schedule should be flexible, and you should acknowledge that some days will probably be harder than others. Not perfection, but consistency is the key.

Finally, give yourself a treat! Give yourself a small treat for your hard work—a soothing bath, a favorite nutritious food, or even an indulgent Netflix marathon—to show your appreciation. Encouraging yourself with the thought of a tasty prize at the end of your Wall Pilates practice will greatly increase your motivation.To put it simply, motivation cultivation and maintenance are continuous processes. On your Wall Pilates adventure, you'll discover that remaining motivated becomes second nature by adding a rhythmic groove, offering yourself prizes, including diversity, setting realistic goals, and establishing connections with others. You'll continue to benefit from your commitment and diligence if you maintain a good outlook!

EXTRA: Diet While Practicing Wall Pilates

Pilates exercises provide many advantages, such as increased mobility, better balance, toned muscles from head to toe, and increased flexibility. Enhancing your body's nutritional intake might augment the advantages of Pilates.

I've created a comprehensive guide on nutrition for Pilates practitioners that covers everything from when to eat to what to eat before and after a class, the value of staying hydrated while working out, and pre- and post-workout snack and meal options.

When to Eat Before Pilates Class

Not only what you eat before a workout matters, but also when you consume it. It is not a good idea to begin your workouts with a substantial, partially digested lunch. Hundreds are not enjoyable after a large dinner, I promise!

While everyone is different when it comes to the ideal time to eat before working out, there are some general rules to follow. Try not to eat anything an hour before your lesson. You could even wish to give yourself two hours to go between meals and your Pilates session. Try varying the timing and food combinations to determine what suits you the best.

What to Eat Before a Pilates Class

If you eat too little right before a Pilates lesson, you could experience dizziness or fatigue. Overeating might make you feel bloated and tired.

When choosing what to eat prior to a Pilates session, bear the following advice in mind:

- Avoid foods like cabbage, onions, lentils, beans, cauliflower, broccoli, and garlic that can make you bloated or gassy.
- Steer clear of heavy or slow-digesting foods.
- Avoid foods that are high in sugar or carbs
- Avoid large meals or greasy foods
- Steer clear of sugar- and carb-rich foods because they will rise and then crash your blood sugar levels, leaving you feeling lethargic.

Rather, prioritize a low-fat lunch or snack that contains some lean protein, complex carbohydrates, and healthy fat. This mixture will help you maintain balanced energy levels and keep you filled up so you can power through the section.

For your early-morning wall Pilates, choose for something light like a banana with nut butter or a small bowl of yogurt topped with berries and nuts.An hour or two prior to your Pilates session, try these nutritious pre-workout snacks and meals:

RECIPE 1

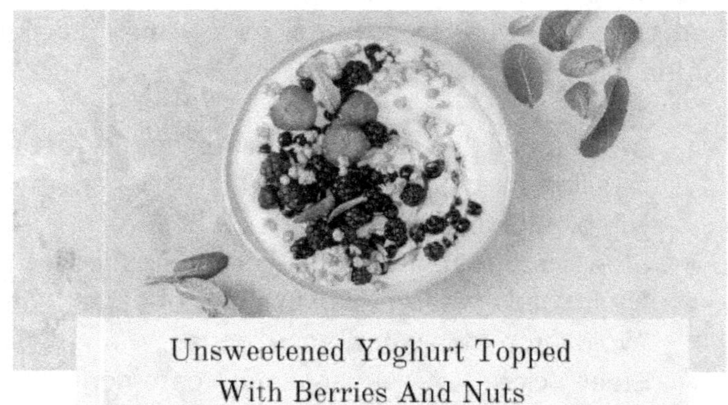

Unsweetened Yoghurt Topped
With Berries And Nuts

PREPPING TIME: 5 MIN   COOKING TIME: 0

Ingredients

- 6 oz nonfat plain Greek yogurt
- 1 tbsp honey, local preferred
- 1/2 cup fresh berries
- 1 tbsp chopped walnuts

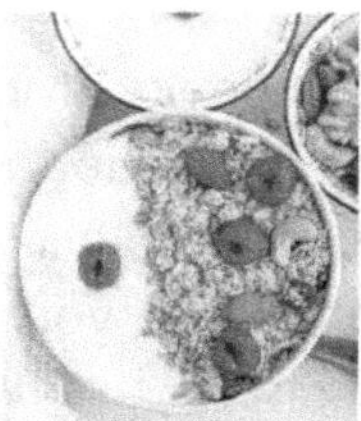

DIRECTION

- Spoon yogurt onto a plate and garnish with honey, nuts, and berries.
- Granola would also be delicious.

RECIPE 2

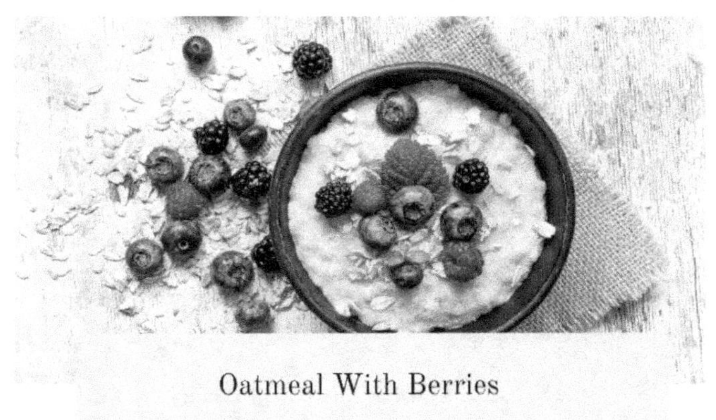

Oatmeal With Berries

PREPPING TIME: 5 MIN   COOKING TIME: 0

Ingredients

- 1/4 Dry rolled oats
- 1/3 Unsweetened low-fat nondairy milk
- Blueberries or berries of choice

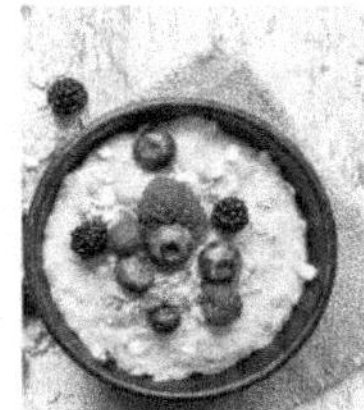

<u>DIRECTION</u>

- Combine oats and low-fat milk in a bowl and place the bowl in the microwave.
- Microwave on HIGH 2-1/2 to 3 minutes.
- Top with berries and yogurt (optional)

RECIPE 3

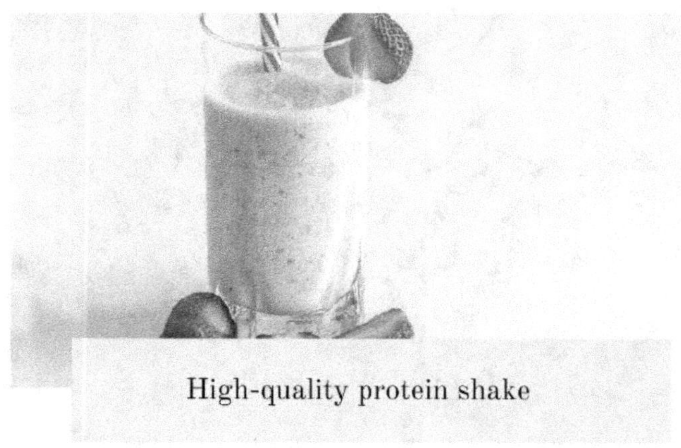

High-quality protein shake

PREPPING TIME: 5 MIN   COOKING TIME: 0

Ingredients

- Milk
- Banana
- Strawberries
- Yogurt
- Protein powder

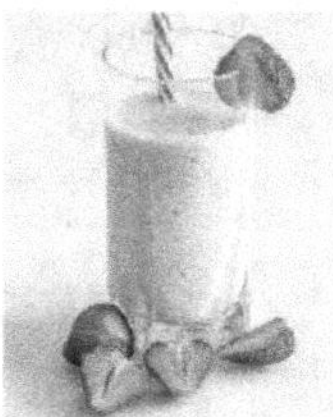

<u>DIRECTION</u>

- Add the ingredients to a blender.
- Blend until smooth and creamy with no chunks of fruit.

When to Eat After Pilates Class

It is crucial that you consume a small meal or snack between 30 and 60 minutes following your Pilates session. This gives your body the lean protein it needs to repair your muscles and replenishes the glycogen stores in your body.

What to Eat After a Pilates Session

You should aim for a mix of complex carbohydrates, healthy fats, and lean protein, much like you would with a pre-workout meal.

Here are a few quick and healthful post-Pilates dinner ideas:

RECIPE 1

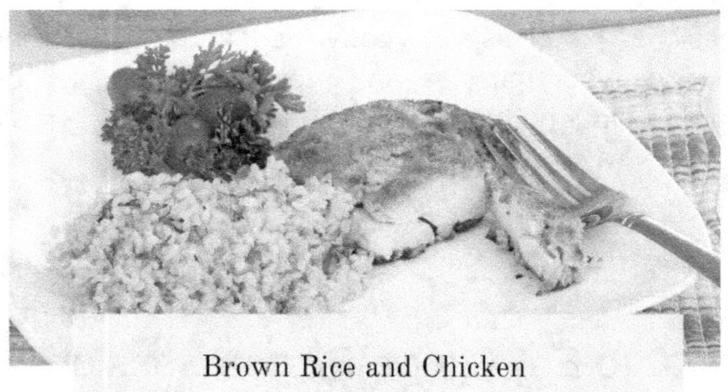

Brown Rice and Chicken

PREPPING TIME: 15 MIN   COOKING TIME: 30

Ingredients

- Vegetable oil
- Frozen peas
- Instant brown rice
- Soy sauce
- Garlic salt
- Eggs
- Matchstick carrots
- Chicken
- Green onion

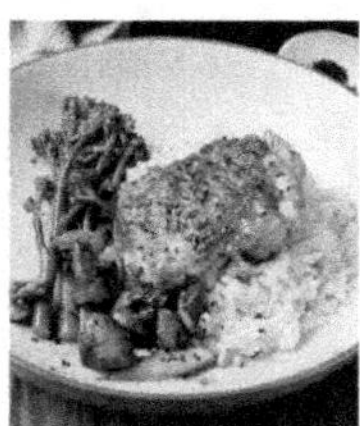

DIRECTION

- Whisk your eggs together.
- Next, add a little oil to a sizable skillet, allow it to get hot, and scramble the eggs over medium heat.

- Once they're scrambled, scrape the eggs out into a bowl and wipe out your skillet.

- Add the chicken with garlic salt and the remaining oil to the same skillet.

- Cook until the center is no longer pink, about medium to medium-high heat.

- Add peas, rice, and soy sauce.

- Cover and cook over medium heat, stirring from time to time, until heated through

- Return the scrambled eggs to the skillet and add carrots, green onions, and remaining soy sauce.
- Stir until well combined and then dig in! You can also serve with sesame oil, soy sauce, hot sauce, and garlic salt if desired

RECIPE 2

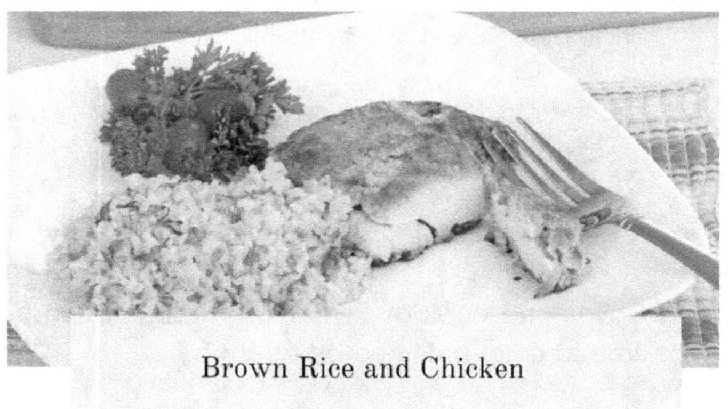

Brown Rice and Chicken

PREPPING TIME: 15 MIN   COOKING TIME: 30

Ingredients

- Vegetable oil
- Frozen peas
- Instant brown rice
- Soy sauce
- Garlic salt
- Eggs
- Matchstick carrots
- Chicken
- Green onion

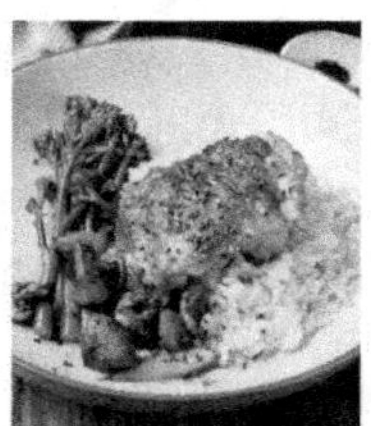

<u>DIRECTION</u>

- Chop and rinse the cabbage and onions. After adding 1 tsp of lemon juice, wait for the eggs to finish boiling. You can skip this step if you'd like. Lemon juice takes away the sharp taste of onions and the potent aroma of cabbage.

- Place them in a mixing basin with the chiles and chopped carrots. Mix well.

- Cube the eggs into the appropriate sizes. Because my kids dislike mushy yolks in their egg salad, I don't slice it extremely small. After adding half of the eggs, season with salt, pepper, and chaat masala.

- Place the remaining vegetables and eggs on top. Add chopped parsley or coriander leaves. Add a little extra virgin olive or virgin coconut oil and pepper powder.

- Toss the salad carefully, covering the bowl. Boiled egg salad is ready and tastes delicious and healthful. It's preferable to serve this right away.

What to Eat In Between Pilates Workouts

Your goals and unique body type will determine what you eat in between Pilates sessions. You may develop strong, lean muscles and maintain steady energy levels by adhering to a balanced diet, which will ensure that you are always prepared for your next workout.

Eat a diet high in whole, nutrient-dense foods, such as:

- Nuts, seeds, and nut butter
- Healthy fats from wild-caught fish (sardines, salmon, tuna, anchovies)
- Unsweetened yogurt
- Fruits
- Vegetables
- Leafy greens

Remember that everything should be done in proportion, so try not to restrict your diet too much. Incorporate a fine dessert every now and again to keep things in check and guarantee long-term success.

Importance of Hydration

Drinking enough water throughout your Wall Pilates exercises is like giving your body a revitalizing sip. It's about nourishing your muscles, increasing your flexibility, and getting the most out of every movement in addition to simply satisfying your thirst.

Imagine yourself performing a sequence of Wall Pilates exercises, your muscles burning, when a gentle nudge to gulp some water appears. It's a time for refueling, not just a rest. During these workouts, staying hydrated is essential to maximizing your performance and general well-being.

Let's start by talking about energy. Your vitality might be drastically reduced by dehydration, which makes you feel worn out and less inclined to put forth your best effort. Having a well-hydrated physique guarantees that you can perform wall sits, leg lifts, and planks with enthusiasm. That water bottle contains all of your natural energy reserves.

Consider flexibility now. Pilates is based on deliberate, fluid movements that work different muscle groups. Drinking enough water lubricates your muscles and joints, making your movements more fluid. Your body will appreciate the increased hydration while you perform those Wall Pilates routines with grace, enabling more effective and graceful movements.

cramping in the muscles? Not when we're watching. Staying well hydrated aids in avoiding uncomfortable muscular cramps and spasms, which can seriously ruin your Pilates practice. Drinking enough water helps your muscles stay flexible and responsive, which lowers your risk of cramping and guarantees that you can perform your exercise with correct form.

Furthermore, the body's natural detoxification process is aided by enough hydration. Not only are you burning calories when performing Wall Pilates movements, but you're also getting rid of pollutants. After a workout, drink plenty of water to help your kidneys eliminate these toxins and feel renewed and invigorated.Let's talk about endurance last. Your best tool for weathering those longer, more difficult Pilates classes is hydration. Your body can better control its temperature when you're hydrated, which helps you avoid overheating and push through your workout without experiencing exhaustion or overheating.

Thus, the next time you set up your mat for a session of Wall Pilates, don't forget to have that water bottle handy. It's more than simply a workout partner—it's your hydration ally, helping you work at your best, move gracefully, and emerge from the session feeling energized and successful. Drink plenty of water and watch the Pilates miracle happen!